praise for
GUIDING stråla

"*Guiding Strala* is the essential handbook to lead from a place
of grace, ease, and effectiveness."
— **DEEPAK CHOPRA,** *New York Times* best-selling
author of *You Are the Universe*

"In *Guiding Strala*, Tara Stiles generously shares the deep principles of the
Strala Yoga lifestyle, thus inviting students, teachers, and leaders on a
joyous journey toward more ease—in both body and mind."
— **JAMES REDFORD,** writer, producer, and director for film and television,
and co-founder and chair of The Redford Center

"This book provides an exciting and impeccable road map for leaders of all backgrounds and
pursuits. And it gives a clear process we can readily embody, for releasing tension and getting
back into the flow . . . Whether you're leading a yoga class or a business, supporting your team
or your family, *Guiding Strala* will uplift and enable your life, in everything you do."
— **RUDOLPH E. TANZI, PH.D.,** *New York Times* best-selling
author of *Super Brain* and *Super Genes*

"*Guiding Strala* is the foundational guidebook for anyone looking to use
movement as a tool to live a better, happier, and healthier life."
— **JASON WACHOB,** founder & CEO of mindbodygreen
and author of *Wellth*

"Tara's book illuminates a clear path for anyone with a call to lead themselves
and others into a rewarding journey of joy and radiant well-being."
— **GABRIELLE BERNSTEIN,** #1 *New York Times* best-selling
author of *The Universe Has Your Back*

"This is a wonderful resource for anyone wanting to bring healing and well-being
into any aspect of self-care and leadership. I personally love the level
of transformation the practice of Strala brings."
— **JESSICA ORTNER,** *New York Times* best-selling
author of *The Tapping Solution for Weight Loss and Body Confidence*

"*Guiding Strala* is full of practical wisdom on how to lead with ease and experience life
from a place of deep peace. In incorporating Strala into my own practice, I found a deeper
mind-body connection, and the confidence to explore the full potential for happiness and
health. Tara's insights will enable readers to transform their lives from the inside out."
— **BARB SCHMIDT,** co-founder of the movement Peaceful Mind Peaceful Life
and international best-selling author of *The Practice*

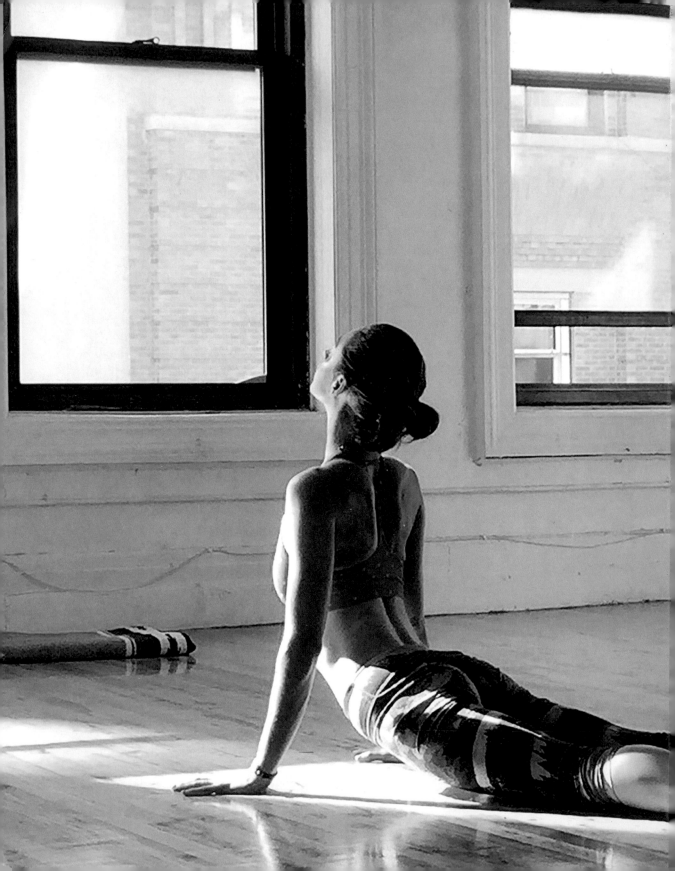

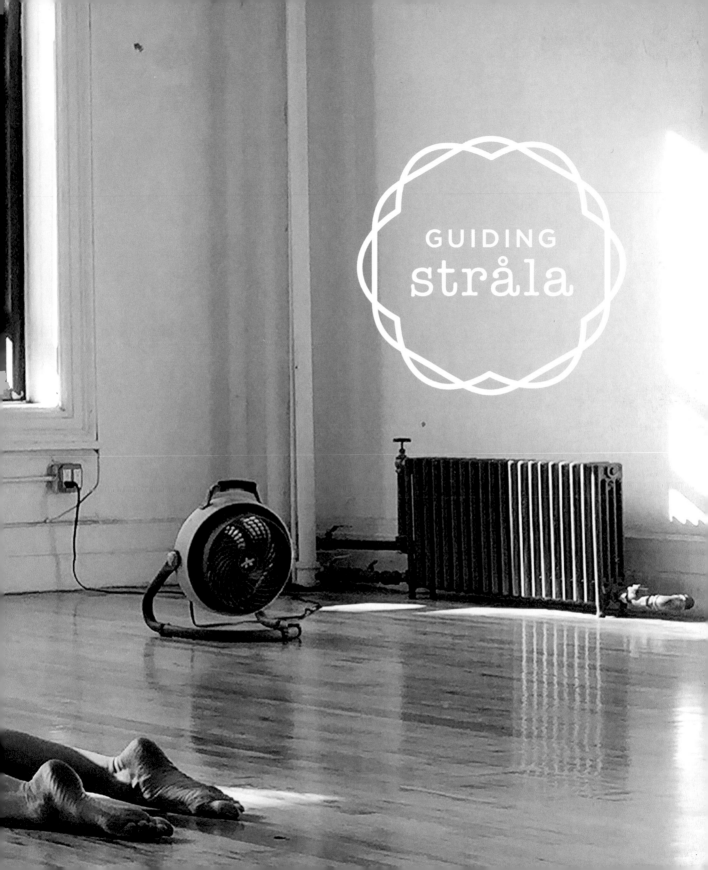

GUIDING
stråla

GUIDING
stråla

THE YOGA TRAINING MANUAL

TO IGNITE FREEDOM,
GET CONNECTED,
AND BUILD RADIANT
HEALTH AND
HAPPINESS

TARA STILES

HAY HOUSE, INC.
Carlsbad, California • New York City • London
Sydney • Johannesburg • Vancouver • New Delhi

Published and distributed in the United States by: Hay House, Inc.: www.hayhouse.com® •
Published and distributed in Australia by: Hay House Australia Pty. Ltd.: www.hayhouse.com.au •
Published and distributed in the United Kingdom by: Hay House UK, Ltd.: www.hayhouse.co.uk •
Published and distributed in the Republic of South Africa by: Hay House SA (Pty), Ltd.:
www.hayhouse.co.za • *Distributed in Canada by: Raincoast Books:* www.raincoast.com •
Published in India by: Hay House Publishers India: www.hayhouse.co.in

Indexer: Jay Kreider • *Book design:* Charles McStravick
Interior photos: Photo of Rudolph Tanzi on page x by Jeremiah Sullivan •
Photo of Kayleigh Pleas on page 18 by Mikal McAllister •
Yoga routine photos courtesy of Thomas Hoeffgen •
Photo on page vi under license from Shutterstock.com •
All other photos courtesy of Tara Stiles

Library of Congress Cataloging-in-Publication Data

Names: Stiles, Tara, author.
Title: Guiding Strala : the yoga training manual to ignite
freedom, get connected, and build radiant
health and happiness / Tara Stiles.
Description: 1st Edition. | Carlsbad :
Hay House, Inc., 2017. | Includes index.
Identifiers: LCCN 2016057824 | ISBN 9781401948108
(tradepaper : alk. paper)
Subjects: LCSH: Yoga. | Mind and body. | Self-care, Health.
Classification: LCC RA781.7 .S748 2017 | DDC 613.7/046--dc23 LC
record available at https://lccn.loc.gov/2016057824

Tradepaper ISBN: 978-1-4019-4810-8

10 9 8 7 6 5 4 3 2 1
1st edition, May 2017

SUSTAINABLE
FORESTRY
INITIATIVE

Certified Chain of Custody
Promoting Sustainable Forestry
www.sfiprogram.org
SFI-01268

SFI label applies to the cover stock

PRINTED IN THE UNITED STATES OF AMERICA

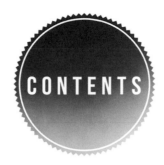

CONTENTS

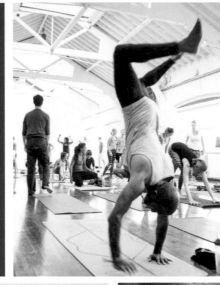
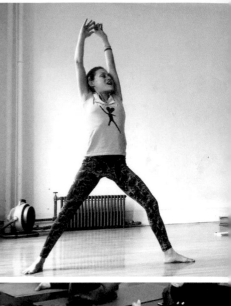
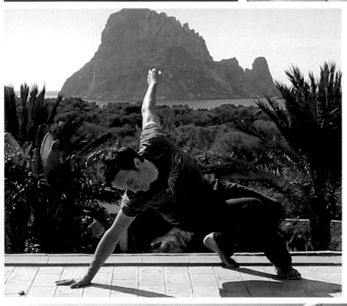
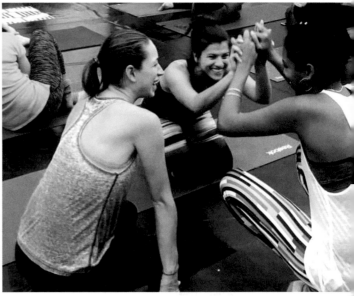
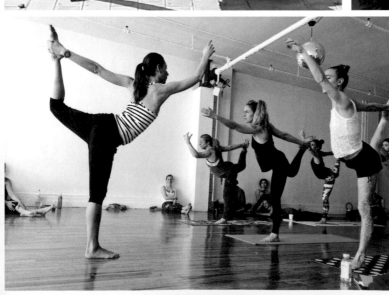

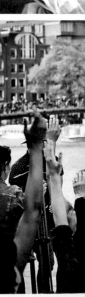

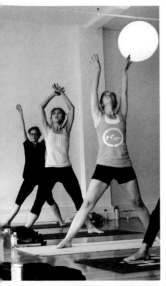
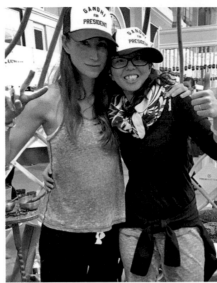
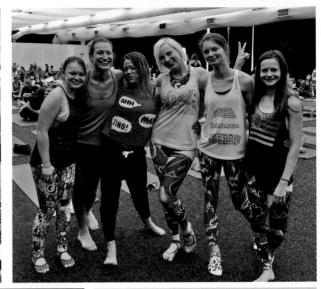
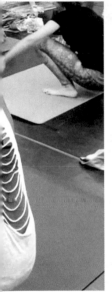
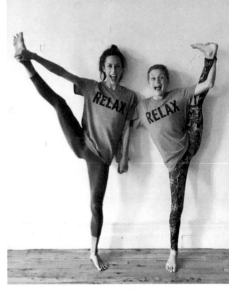

> "It's not the yoga that heals you.
> It's you that heals you."

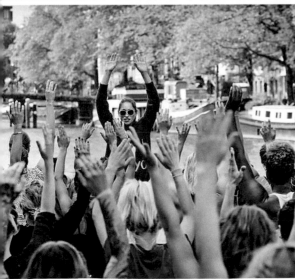
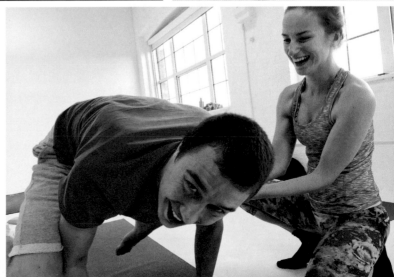

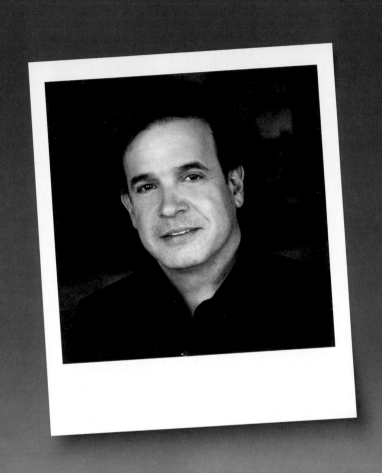

FOREWORD

BY RUDOLPH E. TANZI, Ph.D.

In the last 20 years, we've made some astonishing discoveries. We know now that our neurological makeup is dynamic and plastic, every day re-created in response to how we each move through our lives. We know that our genetic activity, called gene expression, is also soft-wired, not hardwired, equally responsive to our daily activity. And we know more than ever that stress, both physical and emotional, is central to the ailments we struggle with most. It leads to faster aging, obesity, anxiety and depression, autoimmune and digestive disorders, chronic pain, heart disease, cancer, and neurological disorders. Stress also produces chronic inflammation, which compromises many of our body's critical systems, and plays a key role in Alzheimer's disease.

Maybe most important in all this: we know that we are each in the driver's seat of our own lives, in control of our personal destiny. We know we can change our own health, and our entire life experience—on chemical, neurological, and genetic levels—through the choices we make each day. Our lives are our own to create.

So how do we get on this path to creating what we want? Many modern approaches to fitness and self-care actually increase our stress burden, often in an attempt to address what we see as wrong with our bodies. Since stress isn't a sustainable health system, this might not be our best strategy.

Strala is a powerful and revolutionary approach to self-care that decreases our stress burden, supports what's right with our bodies, and leads to astonishing levels of both health and fitness. It accomplishes this in two steps.

First, Strala gives us a keen sense of perspective, a mind-set that readily disposes the stress-inducing attitude of no pain no gain, replacing it with something that works much better. Strala allows us to realize that we can accomplish far more in our bodies, and in our lives, by feeling good every step of the way, by becoming whole in body, mind, and spirit. The resulting sense of balance and harmony carries us further than aggression, right down to the level of our nervous system and genes.

Second, Strala gives us a breath and movement practice, which puts our bodies and minds where they need to be in order to do away with suffering and foster healing. It puts our destiny in our own hands, catapulting us beyond our dreams. This practice allows us to let go of struggle, find inner balance, and move with grace and coordination in everything we do. Most importantly, it teaches us how to release stress and tension from our minds and our bodies, no matter what challenges we face. We find ourselves more flexible and adaptable not only in body, but in mind and spirit. In this way, we're able to create the body and mind we need, to thrive in this world.

I've had access to all kinds of yoga, and all kinds of approaches for handling stress and illness. There are many possible benefits, but also some common missing elements. And when it comes to yoga, most of what's missing is connected to a pattern of rigidity, that limits the potential of yoga to heal and enable us. In fact, nearly every mental illness can be categorized either by the presence of chaos, or rigidity. So when we find rigidity in yoga—in our healing practices—we know it's time to make a change. What I love about Strala is it creates this change by making us free to live dynamic and infinitely adaptable lives, in which mental and physical well-being reciprocally strengthen each other on a daily basis.

The key is to release ourselves from stress and the prison of rigidity, learning to live a different way. We have an astonishing power to rewire our bodies and minds, through how we choose to live. The result is that we end up accomplishing much more, creating the ideal conditions to promote self-healing on all levels.

What I've experienced in Strala is that this system gets it right. It fills in the missing elements. Strala is a highly effective self-care method for releasing the tension that inhibits our health and our lives, on every level that matters, right down to our neural networks and programs of gene expression. I've seen how it also allows us to accomplish far more, by creating a new physical reality of who we are. It's an elegantly simple and sophisticated way to move our breath, our body, and our whole self into the state we need, to create who we want to be: the optimal expression of ourselves.

Guiding Strala provides an exciting and impeccable road map for leaders of all backgrounds and pursuits. It gives a clear process we can readily embody, for releasing tension and getting back into the flow. We learn to mobilize and empower ourselves through a mind-set and practice that leads to accomplishing more with less effort. And most importantly, we form a positive connection with our most radiant self, which, in turn, allows us to form a positive connection with the people around us. Whether you're leading a yoga class or a business, supporting your team or your family, *Guiding Strala* will uplift and enable your life, in everything you do.

My own work led to *Super Brain,* then *Super Genes.* Strala leads us to a Super Self, which enriches the lives of all around us. The more people incorporate the practices of *Guiding Strala* into their everyday lives, the more relaxed, inspired, and uplifted our world will become. The physical and mental freedom gained from Strala allows us to maximally enjoy our own existence while enhancing that of those around us. And it all begins with what we can visualize and create, within each and every one of us. Let Strala guide your way.

— **RUDOLPH E. TANZI, PH.D.,**
New York Times best-selling author of *Super Brain* and *Super Genes*

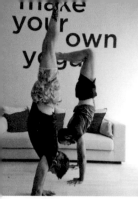

make
your
own
yoga

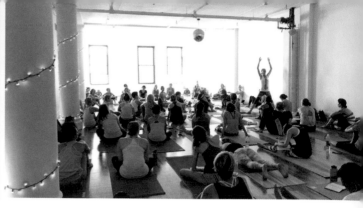

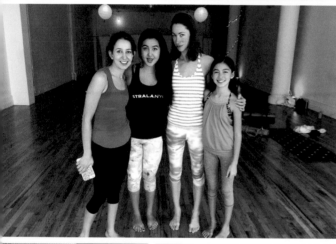

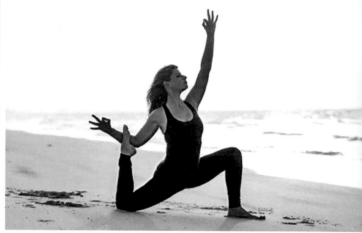

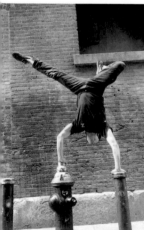

> "
> Ultimately we give others
> the experience of how we feel
> about ourselves.
> "

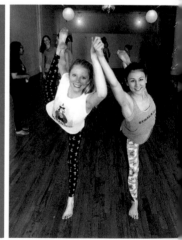

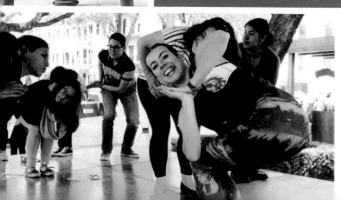

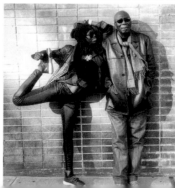

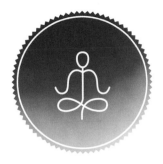

INTRODUCTION

Welcome to Strala—and, more specifically, *Guiding Strala!* I'm thrilled you're here. I'm also energized by your desire to live with ease and your passion to inspire others to do the same. And I'm not going to lie; your dedication to leading a wellness revolution makes me hopeful for our future.

Whether or not you realize it, you are already a leader. Everyone is. Everyone leaves impressions on other people simply through their actions and how they interact with the world. But what you are doing now is trying to take it up a notch—to become a *great* leader. To do this, you need not only a wealth of experience, an ocean of knowledge, and an ability to inspire but also, perhaps most valuable, a mastery of the self.

The first step in this quest is becoming aware of how your actions and outlook affect your own life and the lives of those around you. Since you're here, I suspect you understand this. You understand the words above: ultimately we give others the experience of how we feel about ourselves. To truly lead well, we must embody the principles and practices we're trying to teach. This is an integral part of the journey you're on.

The other piece of becoming a great leader is to make the brave decision to consciously lead, to share what you know in a structured manner. In this case, you have chosen to become a Strala Guide. I'm so glad to be on this exciting journey with you.

My goal is to empower you to lead others to an easeful experience of life. Through the physical, mental, and emotional practice of Strala Yoga, you can teach people how to achieve more with less effort, conserve energy, and become aware of themselves and the world around them, and in turn become more healthy, happy, and radiant.

This practice is inarguably relevant for our lives in this insanely fast-paced day and age. We have endless amounts of information at our fingertips. We're constantly short on time, rushed, and frantic. Our to-do lists never seem to get smaller. We are stressed beyond belief. In fact, stress is currently the largest crisis of the human race. It's a major cause of sickness and disease, and it's a huge factor in creating a disconnection between our bodies and our minds. Once this disconnection sets in, our frazzled minds become programmed to search for the quick fix for whatever symptom ails us in the moment. We gobble up a fast-food meal to deal with our hunger. We down a pill or a drink to help with our anxiety. We always choose something easy at the cost of our well-being.

Sadly much of yoga has evolved to mirror the problems we experience in modern society. It promotes disconnection by encouraging extreme movements and intimidating poses. It inspires stress and competition through a focus on perfect alignment and pushing toward goals. And it often ends in injury and pain. Without meaning to, we've created a practice of stress and frustration rather than peace and contentment.

I like to think of Strala Yoga as the antithesis of modern yoga and modern society. It is about slowing down, softening, and relearning how to move naturally, with the goal of sensitizing ourselves to how we feel and connecting with our bodies. It guides us to focus on the process. It's not about perfecting a pose; it's about choosing our movements based on what's best for us in both the moment and the long term.

Strala is a practice that starts with people—just as they are right now. It is designed to work for people of any age, any background, any body type, and any level of experience. Everyone can practice, and because of this, the group experience of Strala is wonderfully diverse. And the experience of guiding Strala is beyond rewarding.

All the ancient texts remind us that yoga is an inside job. It's about practicing in order to experience our true nature of well-being and oneness. This is what Strala Yoga aims to do. And from what I've experienced in my own life—and seen in the lives of other practitioners—it works. Living this way promotes radiant health and happiness, and most exciting for our modern lives, it dissolves stress.

EXPERIENCE & ORCHESTRATE

Guiding Strala is a leader's handbook that explores the principles and practices of Strala so you can bring them to others. The concepts apply to how we are in our bodies and minds, how we move, how we practice, and how we guide others to create lasting change in their own lives. These principles relate not only to guiding a yoga class but also, more broadly, to a lifestyle of radical well-being.

The book is set up to go along with the belief that you must embody to lead. In Part I Mike Taylor, Sam Berlind, and I (the core Strala faculty), along with frequent guest Kayleigh Pleas, take you through the philosophies of Strala and help you experience them in your own life. *Experience* is the heart of what you'll share when you're guiding others. To be an effective Guide, it's important to be excellent at what you're leading. It's not something you turn on when you lead class and turn off when it's over. You are essentially sharing who you are with others. So you must first get loads of practice so you are acting from a place that is authentically you.

Gaining more and more experience will also take care of many of the little questions and quirks and hiccups of leading. Common problems with the timing of the class, pacing of the sequences, and getting people to follow along, be relaxed, and accomplish the movements with ease can be solved by going back to your firsthand knowledge of what works and what doesn't.

In Part II we focus on the logistics of taking this information beyond you—we help you learn to lead Strala. Basically, we teach you how to orchestrate a class. *Orchestrating* is the approach and technique of leading. It's the how, what, where, and all the ins and outs of taking people through a class. It's attitude, body position, language, mirroring, use of voice, demonstrating, touch, and support. We cover everything it takes to create a welcoming environment and an inspiring class that will positively impact the people who take it. There is a switch of gears that happens when you move from *experience* to *orchestrate*. It is the change from considering yourself to considering others. It's critical to consider these two phases to be an effective Guide. You need to be simultaneously in tune with yourself and able to look beyond yourself.

Then finally in Part III, we move beyond the mat and look at other areas of life that often work their way into the process of guiding a wellness program: eating well and creating a life based on passion.

Before you dive into the pages, I suggest that you gather just a few things. First, you should get a journal. This is handy for writing down your thoughts, ideas, and what inspires you. You'll need some comfortable clothes that you can freely move around in to practice, and some open space and a mat would be good too. For the work you'll be doing in Part II, you'll need to gather some people. Remember, this process is about learning how to guide, which means you need some students to give you experience. So get the living room ready for friends and family to enjoy your classes and support. If you have someone else in your life who would be interested in guiding, grab that training buddy to go through the material with you and work together as Guides. Having a partner to practice on is incredibly useful, and the feedback you can give each other is invaluable.

This book is designed to accompany a Strala training program, which you can find happening around the world. It is not a substitute for in-person training; it's a reference that will support you as you begin to practice and lead.

The reason I've designed this information as a book that's available to anyone—rather than a secret training manual exclusively handed down from person to person—is to give anyone the tools and confidence to help those around them. As I mentioned before, we are all leaders, whether we mean to be or not, so the more you know, the better off the world is.

Thank you for coming along for the ride and for all the good you do in the world. We need you to rise and lead so we can experience lasting, sustainable change. Embody and share what inspires you. Alone we can help a few. Together we can serve the world.

Serve with love.

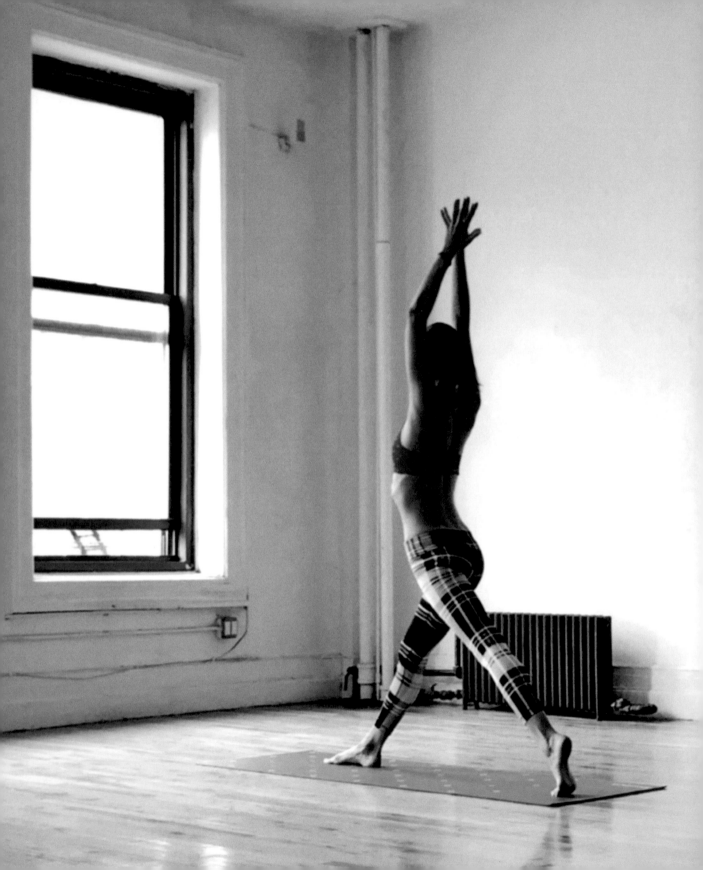

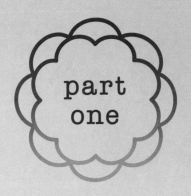

part
one

experience

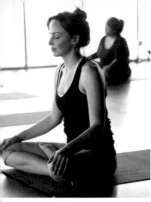

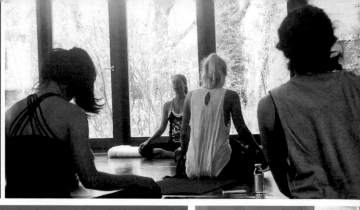
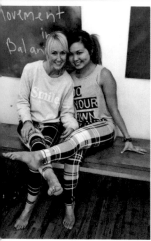

> How you practice anything
> is how you are at
> everything.

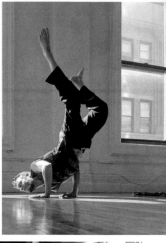
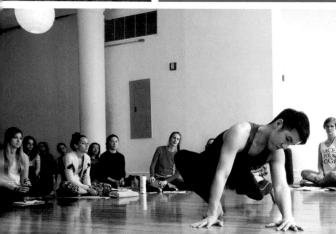
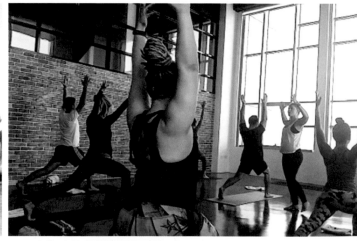
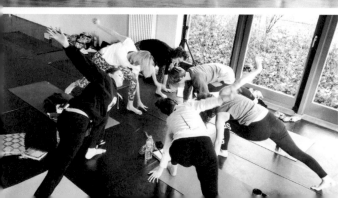
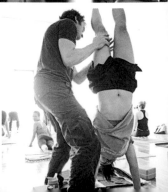

chapter
1

YOGA & EASE

THE STRALA PHILOSOPHY

The philosophy of Strala Yoga was inspired by the experiences I had growing up on a farm in Illinois. Without planning to do so, I started a self-taught practice of yoga and meditation using nature to connect, enjoy, and get excited about my life's purpose. I would sit comfortably, close my eyes, and connect inward. I would move with the wind and flow with the water. I let nature infect my thoughts and my body—and when I did this I felt a profound and energizing sense of space, calm, and excitement for my life's possibilities. I also felt a strong desire to serve and help others. I loved dreaming about how amazing the world could be.

As I moved through life, I slowly started getting away from this natural state of connection and joy. I got busy. I got stressed. I got caught up in the to-ings and fro-ings of life. And soon enough I started to feel sick and unhappy. Just a lack of energy all around. Life was hard—and it wasn't simply because I was an adult with adult responsibilities. Life was hard because that was my mind-set. I thought I had to work hard to succeed. And I worked hard. And then harder. And harder yet.

But after some time of suffering, I began to look within. I came to realize that living a joyful life rested in living a life of ease. I don't mean an easy life. I mean a life where you tap into yourself so you can understand just where you are and how best to move forward. It's not about forcing yourself in predetermined directions or fighting for everything you want. Ease is the basis of expansion, growth, healing, and innovation. An approach of ease can take you to—and even beyond—your goal without taxing your spirit or ruining your health.

We've been taught that ease is the path of laziness. Society tells us we need to push through pain to get anywhere good, so we turn off our natural wisdom and trick ourselves in an effort to achieve in a way that others prescribe. In this world, people who are stressed, tense, and unhealthy are held up as good examples. You must work hard, accomplish tasks, and trudge on. Being calm and connected and feeling good is okay only as a reward. You have to earn that vacation or retirement with years of punishment. This may sound harsh, but it's the truth of how we live.

Even in healing practices themselves, pain, tension, and simmering in stress and sadness has been glorified. Instead of tuning in to the effects of these practices, we concentrate on how good we are at them. Instead of allowing them to be a tool to improve our lives, we implement them as a constricting, judgment-filled achievement. Pushing deeper and applying tension and force has desensitized us from our own sense of reason and taken us through a wild storm of chaos masked in the language of healing.

It's against everything we learn (not everything we know) to back away from tension and stress and seek a better way. We need to spend some time reconnecting with our own wisdom, brewing in the practice of working in an easygoing manner. I'm not asking for you to believe in anything, change your religion, or even change your habits; I'm asking you to do yourself the biggest favor of your life. Take a step forward in believing in yourself—not in what society has taught you.

The system of Strala is a practice and philosophy of yoga and healing concentrated on moving naturally and mindfully. The basis of Strala is ease. Ease isn't a destination; it's a journey. It's fundamentally a way of being, moving, and healing that reminds us to use less effort, move naturally, follow our intuition, and allow space for our bodies and minds to build strength, healthy mobility, and radiant well-being.

EASE

NOUN

1. Absence of difficulty or effort.

2. Freedom from labor, pain, or physical annoyance; tranquil rest; comfort.

VERB

1. Make (something unpleasant, painful, or intense) less serious or severe.

2. Move carefully, gradually, or gently.

The laws of Strala are the laws of nature; they are nothing new, but they can be radical when put into practice. Movements in Strala are slow, steady, and continuous. Tension and anxiety dissolve and have no chance of accumulating with this fluid approach. Focus is on the process, not the goal. It's about softly expanding our comfort zone, which in turn takes us to our goal. We access our bodies' wisdom by prioritizing exploration, moving into places that feel good, and backing away from pain.

Self-care lands at the center of a practice of ease. We have to choose to let the work be easygoing as we stay in the process. By doing so, hard things become easy; our health is restored; we get connected to intuition and creativity; and we experience improved focus, attention, and concentration.

A lot of the feedback after Strala classes sounds like this: "I feel free to move how it feels good to me." "I never felt so graceful doing challenging moves." "That felt easy, but I know it wasn't easy, because I'm drenched in sweat!" This feedback is fun, exciting, and refreshing because it means people had an easy-going experience. They feel as if a weight has been lifted. They have been liberated from expectations, and they are comfortable and relaxed in the process of movement.

The opportunity in the practice of Strala is approaching both the simple and challenging moments with ease.

TAKING IT EASY

So how do we get to ease? As I said before, ease isn't a destination; it's a process. It's a way of living. The process of ease is the how of doing anything. It doesn't matter what you're doing. How you approach things will make them hard or easy. Approaching with a how of ease can solve a lot of problems. So let's look at the three steps of an easy approach.

STEP 1: **SLOW DOWN.** We move quickly and rigidly without thinking. We need to get somewhere; we hold our breath, clench, work really hard, and hurry up to get there. We leave one destination and race to another, moving further away from ourselves. So how do we remedy this? Slow down. This gives us the space and time to explore possibilities.

STEP 2: **BREATHE DEEPLY.** After opening some space by slowing down, take a big, full, deep breath, and keep them going. Breathing deeply and fully is our lighthouse to sensitizing ourselves to how we feel. When we breathe deeply, we listen to the cues coming from our bodies and our minds. We learn what is going on inside, so we are in an informed position to act positively. Without the breath, we have no space for informed decisions.

STEP 3: FEEL. Feeling is the final fantastic part of ease. After slowing down, creating the space, and breathing deeply, we are now in a position to feel and then respond to how we feel. Without feeling, we are simply doing, like robots, the tasks of our days, or the poses in our yoga classes. We are reacting to external forces rather than responding from a place of intelligence.

Feeling is how we accomplish ease. When we feel, we move easily and make decisions that heal our lives. Prioritizing feeling is the best gift you can give to yourself and everyone around you. If we don't feel, we simply follow what we think we should do. We're located only in our minds, copying the actions of those we've seen before. There is zero space for your own unique body and mind. Without feeling, we do not flourish. We do not express our true selves. Living with ease, we open our lives up to authentic, expansive expression of our true selves.

The three-step process of ease works not only in yoga but in every aspect of life. How do you work on a project you're frustrated with? Slow down, breathe, feel. How do you treat yourself better and break some bad health habits? Slow down, breathe, feel.

When you get into the process of ease, you're on the right path to make great choices and feel great. When you work through challenges with all kinds of tension, you might achieve your goal, but you'll be stressed, tense, and narrow-sighted during your process. You get more with ease than you do with tension. I know that might seem crazy, but ease is much more natural than tension. If you don't believe me, go check out the ocean; watch the waves move naturally with ease. They don't hesitate and tighten when the storm is coming. They roll right along in the most natural path. A tree doesn't freak out when the wind blows. It simply moves its branches to go along for the ride—and, after the storm, the tree remains.

let's practice

You can practice the three steps to ease in many circumstances. Try it out when you're feeling stuck or tense anytime of day. Think of it as a reset to coming back to feeling great and redirecting your efforts toward positive action. When we deal with "the how" of ourselves, "the what" becomes much clearer, simpler, and tension-free.

Let's bring it into a simple movement phrase to experience.

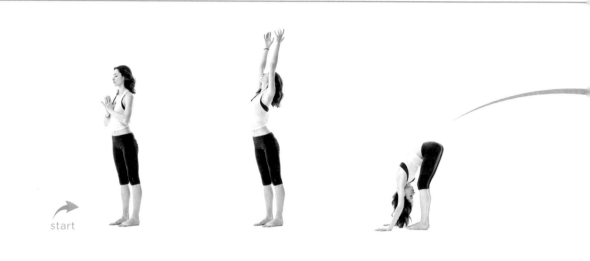

start

Stand tall, steady, and comfortable. Press your palms together, bring your thumbs to your heartbeat, and close your eyes. Widen your feet a bit to have a sturdy stance, and soften your knees. Let your attention drift inward. Allow yourself to shift and drift a bit side to side or forward and back, and soften here for a moment. *Here we are slowing down. Can you feel it? Enjoy it!*

Take a big inhale and lift your arms out and up overhead. Exhale and soften your torso over your legs. *Making some room for those deep breaths to happen. Can you feel it? Enjoy it!*

Soften your knees, press your fingertips on the ground, and step your left leg back to a low lunge. Soften your hips and sway a bit side to side if that feels great for you. *Here we are feeling our way into it. By feeling into the movement, you're exploring around and seeing what's going on with your body. You're expanding your area of possibility from checking*

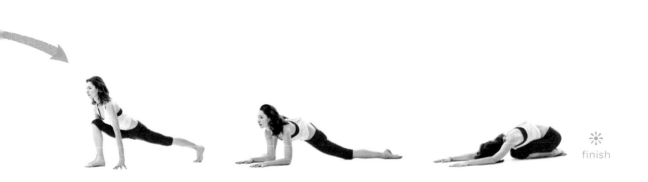

off the pose of low lunge to checking in with how you feel. You're creating a healthy range of mobility in your hips and sensitizing your entire self to feeling great. Relaxation response is kicking in!

Soften your back knee to the ground, and move your front foot out to your side a bit to create some room for your hips. Take a big, deep breath here. Either stay upright if this feels like a lot going on in your hips, or soften your elbows and lower down a bit if that feels nice. Move slowly so you can find a great place to breathe for a while. Hang here for a few long, deep breaths. *Now we are putting it all together. Feels pretty awesome, right?*

When you're ready, lean to your left and slide your front foot around behind you and relax in child's pose for a few long, deep breaths. When you're ready, give it a go on the other side and enjoy!

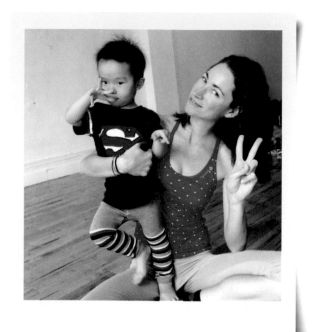

We spend so much time pushing, forcing, and struggling our way through life and even through yoga practice. It's time to stop. It's groundbreaking to realize that how you practice anything is how you are at everything. When we work our bodies and minds in an agitated, frazzled way, we become more agitated and frazzled in our lives. When we begin to participate in the process of ease, we begin to pay attention to our inner wisdom. When we support that with a regular physical practice, our awareness sharpens, intuition expands, and physical strength and a healthy mobility show up to be the best carrier for our whole self. We automatically shine brighter and influence others positively, stirring a desire for self-care in anyone within distance to catch the vibe.

THE PIECES OF STRALA

While the general outlook of Strala is all about ease, we define Strala in three parts that rely on one another to make a whole. The three parts are being, moving, and healing. You can imagine these in three concentric circles, with being in the middle. Being easeful in life leads to moving in an easeful way, which leads to healing. This circular depiction is a nice symbol of radiating from the inside out.

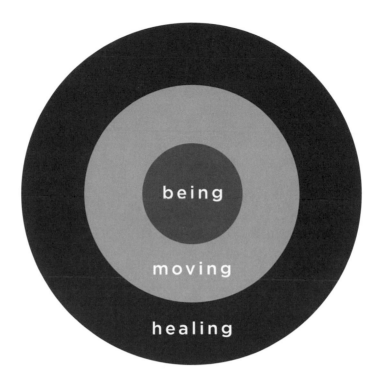

BEING embodies how you are. It's the regular practice that leads to experience and mastery of the Guide. We give what we are, so it's most important to practice improving how we are as long as we're here. Being is the act of prioritizing self-practice to improve our abilities and effectiveness in helping others. Remember, how we do anything is how we do everything.

MOVING embodies how you go about things. It's the process of moving easily, everything you've got in every direction you can. It's moving with ease through simple and challenging moments alike. It's the "how" of the practice. We move naturally, with the least amount of effort, to improve efficiency and promote healing. When we move with ease, we strengthen quickly and effectively, gain a healthy range of mobility, and open room for the attention to rest inward, expanding creativity and intuition.

HEALING is what you do with a mastery of being and moving. It's the prize of the practice. When we put our attention on how we are and how we go about things, we gain more skill and confidence to heal ourselves and develop the capacity to help others heal. We practice to heal imbalance; improve immunity; ignite the relaxation response; recover from injury, trauma, and stress; and enjoy lasting well-being. When we are balanced, we have the capacity to help others find their own balance.

UNDERSTANDING THROUGH CONTEXT

To fully understand what makes Strala and this concept of ease so different, I think it's helpful to look at the history of yoga and how it has evolved over the years.

To start, let's look back to 5,000 years ago in the Indus Valley. While we don't have any specific texts explaining lifestyle or belief systems, stone carvings that depict people sitting in meditative-looking positions have been found. Without additional information it's impossible to say exactly what these carvings mean, but many have interpreted them to be depictions of an early form of yoga.

Between 2,500 and 3,500 years ago, we get our first written records of life: the Vedas. These sacred texts are the basis for Hinduism. Yogis at this time were often solitary types who lived in forests. Their interests aimed at enduring physical hardship by sharpening their minds. There was also a great focus on the power of the breath.

We can see one of the first known shifts in yoga in what was called the Pre-Classical period, which started about 2,500 years ago, when the Upanishads were written. The Upanishads are considered by some to be the final chapters of the Vedas. The Bhagavad Gita, which is the oldest known yoga scripture, dating to 500 B.C.E. was also written during this time. With this text yoga practice seems to have softened a bit, becoming more meditative and less reclusive.

Then we get to Patanjali's Yoga Sutras. This text, which defines the Classical period of yoga, outlines something called the Eightfold Path of yoga. It lays out what to do and not do; how to relate with ourselves and others; and how to sit, breathe, withdraw, focus, concentrate, meditate, and, of course, enlighten. It's worth noting that there is only a single mention of physical activity in this text, and it's mentioned as preparation for proper sitting.

The most recent move is into the yoga of today, which is all about movement. We have Iyengar, Ashtanga, Vinyasa, Kundalini, Strala, and so many more! Yoga likely came to the United States in the 1800s, but its popularity really emerged in the 1960s. Along with LSD and trips to India.

So why does all this matter? It's because context gives us a constant that ties all these different types of yoga together. The one constant for yoga, throughout all its changes over all this time, is that it has always made sense right where it is. It has always been about opening up our minds and helping us tap into that space inside through whatever physical practice was called for at the time.

Five thousand years ago in the Indus Valley, everyone was farming. People worked hard on their feet, and they moved around quite a lot. Whether we call those stone carvings yoga or not, it makes sense that people needed to sit down and rest. Sitting and getting quiet has a way of uncovering some interesting things.

Moving along to 2,500 years ago: this was when we came in from the fields and started living in cities—and making one another sick! Respiratory infections abounded during this era, so it makes sense that breathing techniques found their way into yoga practice. Once again, sitting and breathing gives way to more interesting discoveries about how capable we are.

Life is a little different today. Many of us are sitting at desks for hours every day. Then we sit in cars. At home we're sitting in front of another computer or maybe the TV. So we have plenty of sitting in our lives. We also have high-tech food that gives us as much energy as the woolly mammoth gave an entire cave family. So what do we need today from our yoga? We probably need to get up, reconnect with our bodies, and move! Thus, the styles of yoga that are popular today are more physical.

With each major change in yoga throughout history, the inventors created what was exactly right for them, at exactly that time and place. The originators of yoga were not likely concerning themselves with what sort of yoga cavepeople were doing, what clothes they were wearing, or what language they spoke. Originators have a way of creating something that is entirely their own, from the inside out.

THE STRALA STEP

While Strala is part of today's yoga, I like to think of it as the next step in yoga's evolution because of its focus on self-exploration and ease. For the past several decades, emerging new yoga styles directed a tremendous amount of attention in one of two directions: they focused on either history or physicality. Both of these extremes lose the essential element of self. For styles that look at history, practitioners ask questions like, "What would Patanjali do, and how does it apply to what I'm doing?" For styles that are all about the physical, the focus is on weight loss, posing, and competing to be the best.

With all the focus on studying old texts, languages, and customs, doing and creating have slipped from center. An academic focus on yoga makes for great historians and discussers of yoga—it can also inform what you do in your own practice—but if we get stuck in the academic, we become followers rather than originators. Just as if we are focusing only on the physical part of yoga.

Strala aims to move back to exploring the self through the physical and mental pursuit of yoga. Its goal is to help you live a good life by doing things in a way that connects you to yourself rather than in an effort to perfect a pose or reach some outside mind state. Strala helps you transform into your most radiant, intuitive self through the practice of easeful being, moving, and healing. This is quite different from other popular forms of physically focused yoga.

Systems like Iyengar emphasize ideas about universally correct alignment, and focus on manipulating the body into specific physical postures. Strala recognizes that people are unique, with their own individual bodies, histories, and needs, and it guides everyone to discover their own best shape from within.

Ashtanga and Vinyasa move swiftly from pose to pose, stopping in the poses to fix mistakes in alignment that occur when movement is unnatural and awkward. Strala embodies the principles of natural movement, so people remain always in alignment with themselves.

Most modern systems of yoga derived from Ashtanga and Vinyasa have users exert as much effort as possible, even when doing very simple things. The idea is that practitioners must burn through suffering to achieve anything significant. Strala returns us to nature, which never works harder than it needs to. This conservation of energy is the gateway to making the impossible possible.

Slow-moving and static forms of yoga like Yin concentrate on holding poses for a long period of time with the hope of restoration. But immobilizing your body in uncomfortable poses tends to induce stress rather than relieve it. In contrast, Strala uses the principles of soft, natural movement to release stress from the body and mind, even while moving through difficult obstacles. These principles are common in ancient East Asian arts like tai chi, where movement is at once meditation, healer, and a path to great physical and mental ability. Strala returns this richness to yoga.

Kundalini Yoga has a central focus on intense breathing techniques while holding poses for long periods. The aim is to create a state of mind that is outside your normal life to reach transcendence. Strala takes a different approach. Strala aims to sensitize you to a healthy range of feeling and emotion in everything you do, all day, every day. This is accomplished not by transcending or going someplace else but by being fully here, fully connected to yourself.

Many experience benefits and transformations from all styles of modern yoga, and this is wonderful. But I believe that these other forms fall short of what yoga *could* do for us.

THE SCIENCE OF EASE

Living in ease and getting into feeling mode might seem a little spacey, but the truth is that it's essential to thriving in modern society. Science now confirms that setting our bodies and minds at ease helps us heal, restore, repair, and create lasting good health. Staying connected to how you feel, while breathing deep and moving easily in response to this feeling, ignites your relaxation response—a chemical cascade that promotes both healing and well-being. This is where we want to spend most of our time, but too often we get stuck in a stress response—a different chemical cascade designed to help us survive immediate attack. So we need to get unstuck, out of living under attack, and back into feeling good.

When we are stressed—in life or in yoga class—our body creates hormones that allow us to fight or flee at a moment's notice. This is a good state to be in when we are literally in danger and need to hightail it up a tree to avoid a bear, but the problem is that these same chemicals inhibit our digestion and connection to intuition, unbalance our microbiome, make us age faster, and damage our ability to heal. They basically minimize every bodily function that doesn't deal with staying alive in that moment of danger. With all the stress of life today, we bathe in these stress hormones all the time. When we focus on nailing a yoga pose to perfection, or when we have a tough day at the office, our body stays in this survival mode. There's a better way to be, and we can learn how to get there.

How we live each day has a real, concrete, and profound impact on our bodies, our biology, and our lives. We create ourselves—our neural pathways and connections, our gene expression, even what we pass along to our children—in how we move through each day. We are not only our own to discover. We are our own to create.

This is a ground-shaking, earthmoving discovery. We each live in a body that we create in every moment, through the choices we make. We each live in a world that we create in every moment, through the choices we make. And we can choose right now to become our own best caregivers and creators. We can release stress from our minds, and from how we move in our lives. We can heal. We can align with our nature and unblock our energy. And when energy flows, potential and reality become the same.

I have a couple of amazing friends from whom I've learned so much over the years, and whose support has been tremendous in the evolution of Strala. One is Dr. Deepak Chopra, an inspiring pioneer in mind-body medicine and its application to our everyday lives. The other is Dr. Rudolph Tanzi, a neurology professor at Harvard University and director of the Genetics and Aging Research Unit at Massachusetts General Hospital. They were speaking together at a recent Sages & Scientists symposium, and something was said that stuck in my mind: nearly all mental disorders are connected to either chaos or rigidity. Creating our own radiant health and healing is found on a middle path. It has a structure and process that makes progress possible, while maintaining the freedom of self-discovery and direction. Not chaotic, not rigid. Beautifully diverse in our path to a universally connected well-being.

This is why we created Strala. And I'll guess that this art of moving in our lives—softening, connecting, finding your own way in your own body—creates something like fractal geometry. There's a beautiful order to our individuality, connecting us together in a much bigger picture.

It has me thinking also about the rigidity found within most modern yoga—one correct way, one correct look, even rigidly holding tension in every form and movement. We wouldn't usually look for a cure by practicing more of the disorder. So I have to ask: Are these forms an expression of mental illness, accidentally carrying along the same disorders we're seeking to heal?

I'm going to guess that holding rigidity and tension, for most of us, is just practicing what we're already too good at. More stress. It's bringing our most common neurosis into our cure. Maybe this works occasionally and by accident—because our bodies have a way of healing themselves. We're pretty amazing this way. But I think we can all do even better, by letting the stress go and learning to accomplish challenge in a soft, peaceful, and easygoing way. It takes practice. It's very different from the myth we've been taught about what it takes to succeed in this world. You're worth it.

Kayleigh Pleas, who has led classes and workshops for years at the NYC Strala studio, is an amazing example of the power of ease. Being around her and taking her class is a breath of fresh air. You literally feel relaxed just standing or practicing next to her. This isn't a magic act, nor has she been tossed in more fairy dust than the rest of us. She makes it an active practice to enjoy simmering in relaxation.

Kayleigh also has a background in teaching positive psychology, and she does a lot of work with the military and other groups in stress management training. Because of this experience—and her personal story—she does an amazing job of explaining the science of ease. I hope her story and her explanation of the body's stress response will inspire you.

KAYLEIGH:

I spent the first half of my life pushing and striving to be a better version of myself, driven by a ceaseless inner judge. An elite gymnast by the age of 13, I believed "success" meant perfection, and perfection was achieved through struggle. And struggling I was. By my early 20s, I was suffering from insomnia, anxiety, and a stress-related digestive disorder called irritable bowel syndrome (IBS). My life felt like a long to-do list. I was always on my way to the next goal that I hoped would quiet the ever-present fear that I was not good enough. When no acute, physical cause for my digestive troubles could be found, the doctors told me I had low serotonin and prescribed antidepressants.

I walked through the doors of Strala at a turning point. After a lifetime of motivating myself to achieve through harsh criticism and control, I was forced to sit with the truth: my striving was making me sick, and no amount of trying hard could

bring the deep inner contentment I so longed to experience. In the welcoming Strala studio, as I learned to soften and breathe into my movement, my critical mind naturally quieted, and an inner joyfulness I had long forgotten started to emerge. I didn't know what was happening physiologically, but I knew I wanted my life to feel the way I felt doing Strala.

Over the past 11 years, the desire to understand why I had low serotonin grew into a dedication to the study of human well-being—physical, mental, emotional, and spiritual.

I am particularly fascinated by how the mind and body affect each other—and how this interaction can be leveraged for well-being. In a happy coincidence, at the same time I found Strala, I was completing my master's degree in applied positive psychology, researching how the way we motivate ourselves, whether through harsh criticism or kind support, affects the brain and nervous system.

Two important points emerged from my studies: First, I learned that I am not alone in my struggles with self-criticism, stress, and physical-emotional breakdown. We live in a culture with debilitating expectations and messages around who we should be. If we are not happy, we see it as a personal failure and are told to push harder, perfect, and power through. Caught in a tireless pursuit to prove ourselves through controlling and achieving, we end up feeling like something is wrong with us. The CDC estimates that only 17 percent of the adult U.S. population is in a state of optimal mental health. We are a culture suffering from loneliness and self-aggression.

Sadly, as we export the Western way of life around the globe, anxiety and depression continue to rise. The World Health Organization estimates that by 2020, depression will be the second leading cause of disability worldwide. Furthermore, our modern-day health problems (that is, digestive disorders, obesity, insomnia, mental fog, depression, premature aging, diabetes, cancer) are either caused or exacerbated by stress. An estimated 60 to 90 percent of all medical visits are stress related.

Second, I learned why Strala works at the physiological level. Strala is one of the most skillful ways to recalibrate the stress centers of the brain and reclaim an inner motivation and relationship to our bodies and our lives guided by deep care and kindness, as opposed to fear and criticism. When guided to feel our way into our bodies and move because it feels good to move, we reestablish connection with a compassionate part of ourselves that wants to be well. Instead of following a rule about what we should be doing, the body's intelligence guides us to make choices that truly serve happiness and health. Through the practice, we learn to trust ourselves.

Understanding the body's stress response illuminates the power of Strala's philosophy.

When we experience a real or perceived threat, either to one's body (for example, saber-toothed tiger) or sense of self-worth (for example, self-critical thought), the sympathetic nervous system initiates the fight-flight-freeze response, and the body is flooded with the stress hormone cortisol. In the short term, cortisol gives us a jolt of energy and focus. Heart rate and blood pressure increase, breath becomes quick and shallow, and energy is diverted away from the maintenance and repair system of the body to our major muscles. Very helpful when we are running to save our lives!

For our cave ancestors, having a hypersensitive fight-or-flight response was adaptive because threat came in the form of immediate physical danger (for example, saber-toothed tiger crouching in the bushes). Today, facing constant psychological "threats" (related to our perceptions about ourselves, who we should be, and what the future holds), we are living in a state of constant, low-grade sympathetic arousal and running on cortisol until our bodies simply can't take it anymore and we get sick, either physically or mentally.

Think of stress like fire—so powerful it must be used wisely and with control. Left unbridled, stress, like fire, will burn everything in its path. Over time elevated levels of cortisol literally "burn" through muscle, immune, heart, and brain tissues, as well as disrupt the hormonal balance needed for a good mood. The reactive, reptilian part of the brain takes over, and the more recently evolved, wise part of your brain shuts down. Ever wondered why you easily snap at someone you care about when you're stressed? Or have you ever reached for a bag of cookies when you're upset, knowing you didn't want to eat so much sugar? Scientists call this brain state "mild prefrontal cortex dysregulation," which is a fancy term for "blowing your top."

When flooded with cortisol, our thoughts become self-focused and fearful, and our behavior becomes rigid, impulsive, and fear based. We contract into a small, reactive version of ourselves. No time to contemplate what makes life worth living or what you love or to see the beauty around you when your brain thinks you are running from a tiger!

Luckily there's good news! We have the power to intersect the sympathetic nervous system's stress response by activating the rest-and-digest response of the parasympathetic nervous system.

The parasympathetic nervous system is the opposite of the sympathetic nervous system, directing blood and energy back toward the repair and maintenance functions of the body to support digestion, immune function, reproduction, sleep, and the hormones of a good mood. When the overreactive reptilian brain calms down, the wise prefrontal cortex comes back online to broaden our perspective. Seeing clearly, we remember what we care about, what we love, and we guide our actions toward our values.

In Strala we learn to activate the parasympathetic nervous system through both body and mind.

In the body we continuously focus on keeping muscles relaxed. A tense muscle tells the brain that there is danger (tigers abound!); a relaxed muscle tells the brain we are safe (no tigers here). By not focusing on the goal of a pose, we avoid the need to "fix" what we're doing, so we don't tense our muscles and activate the sympathetic wing of our nervous system. By moving with ease, softening, exploring with curiosity, and lingering where it feels good, our muscles relax, and we support parasympathetic dominance.

Long, slow, smooth breathing also tells the brain we are safe. Research demonstrates that a rate of four to six breaths per minute actually arrests the stress response. When we notice and move with the inhalation and exhalation, the breath naturally slows to synchronize to the heart rate.

The bottom line is that a calm body tells the brain that we are safe (no tigers here), which allows the fight-or-flight response to turn off, blood and energy to return to our healing and maintenance systems, and the hormones required for a good mood to flow freely. Amen!

Now let's explore the mind.

The human brain responds to cues in the environment, activating ancient motivation systems that direct physiological processes below conscious control (that is, fluctuating hormone levels, blood distribution, neurotransmitter activity). Two major motivation systems are the threat–self-protection system, which responds to cues of danger or exclusion and evolved to move us away from potential harm, and the soothing/contentment system, which responds to cues of safety and belonging and evolved to bring us together in relationships.

Unfortunately the brain does not differentiate an external cue (a tiger, a warm hug, a bunny rabbit) from an internal cue (a worry, a fond memory, a proud thought). Thus, how we relate to ourselves from moment to moment powerfully affects the neural patterns in the brain and ultimately how we feel about ourselves and the world around us. When we relate to ourselves with criticism and comparison, we activate the threat–self-protection system, which sets off the fight-flight-freeze response and resulting cascade of stress hormones, including cortisol. When we relate to ourselves with kindness and care, we activate the soothing/contentment system, which engages the rest-and-digest response and resulting cascade of feel-good hormones, including the bonding hormone oxytocin.

At Strala, Guides use gentle, supportive language and a warm tone to cue the soothing/contentment system, giving rise to feelings of safety, relaxation, and belonging. When the body's stress response calms and cortisol levels fall, prefrontal cortex functioning improves, leading to greater awareness of thoughts and emotions as merely thoughts and emotions, waves of experience passing through. Here, Strala students come to experience themselves as the steady, ever-present awareness that is beyond the constant monitoring of the ceaseless inner judge.

Over time, as students internalize the supportive voice of the Guide, they start to relate to themselves with the same gentleness off the mat. In daily life, as difficult emotions and thoughts arise, rather than beating themselves up with judgment or numbing through activities like eating, drinking, shopping, or surfing the web, students learn to mindfully attend to the sensations in the body and self-soothe by going inward with kindness. Curiosity about what is happening, deep breathing, and openness to the ever-changing waves of experience become habits of being, which leads to a belief in their inherent value.

For me the work of Strala was beyond expectation. It helped me change a lifetime of critical inner dialogue. As psychologist Paul Gilbert aptly states, "Logic is not enough: 'evidence' is secondary to the experience of being helped and supported." By activating the brain through the body, we can begin to stimulate the various sensations and somatic states needed to elicit the oxytocin response of the soothing system and associated feelings of tenderness and care.

I no longer have IBS, and while I still have my moments of anxiety and self-doubt, I respond to my inner experience with kindness. When the inevitable challenges of life present themselves, rather than pushing and striving, my task is to soften. From this softness, a feeling of connection is born—connection to myself, connection to the moment, connection to those around me, and connection to life itself. I am more courageous and creative than I ever could have imagined—the joy of self-kindness inspires movement toward new challenges and opportunities—not because I need to achieve to feel adequate but because I want to live my most vibrant, happy life!

getting into
feeling mode

Remember, to successfully instruct others to do something, you must embody it in your own life. Let's move through a few simple movements to connect with the breath and tap into feeling. Stay easy and enjoy!

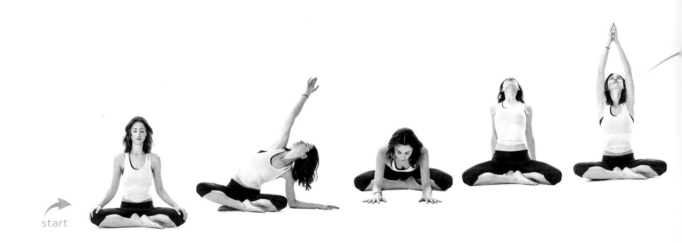

start

Start in a seated position, however you are comfortable. Close your eyes, and rest your attention on your breath. Notice your inhales and exhales as they come and go. Allow yourself to sway side to side and forward and back to find a nice, neutral, balanced place. Settle here for a few moments.

Take a big inhale, and lift your arms up and over your head. Press your palms together, and bring your thumbs to your heartbeat. Soften here for a moment. Take a big inhale through your nose. Long exhale out through your mouth. Twice more just like that. Settle here for a moment.

Lean over toward your left side, reaching your right arm overhead. Roll around here for a bit if that feels nice. Bring yourself back to center and go for the other side. Come back to center and crawl yourself forward. Relax your head and neck and hang here for a few long, deep

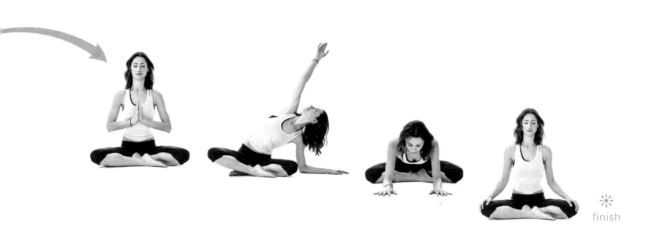

finish

breaths. Bring yourself back upright. Press your hands behind you on the ground for support, take a big inhale, and lift your chest and hips up if that feels good. When you're ready, bring yourself back to seated. Close your eyes, and rest your attention on your breath. Settle here for a few moments. When you're ready, open your eyes.

Now, how do you feel? When you can feel what's going on physically, mentally, and emotionally, you can direct yourself toward empowerment and self-care. When you simmer in this place day after day, you become a magnet for people looking to feel better and grab a little of what you have. But you do need to practice every day. This isn't a one-and-done situation.

WHY WE STRALA

I've been leading Strala formally for more than 10 years now, which honestly seems like no time at all. There are so many stress reactions still left to dissolve in our lives and the world. It's a journey I'm happy to be hunkered down in for the long haul. We all have our own reasons for coming to practice. We practice to be strong, feel confident, be well in our lives, open our creativity, heal from trauma and injury, or connect with our intuition so we can live a fulfilled life. It's critical to consider why we practice so we can dream up a practice that matches.

For me, the desire to help people was inspired by my childhood connection to nature and my self-taught meditation and yoga practices. Once I learned that we can cure so many of our problems by softening our relationship with ourselves, I realized that I needed to help others do this.

I set out on my own personal mission to help anyone who was open to it. If I saw a window of opportunity to help someone feel better, I jumped on it. Opportunity usually came in the form of physical or emotional pain. We can learn a lot from our complaints. What hurts? What are the things we can pinpoint that are holding us back? These things we probably talk about daily. Back pain, anxiety, stress, addiction, lack of confidence, or lack of physical strength. Usually it's not just one complaint but rather a family of destruction. People would complain about aches and pains (which are much easier to talk about than emotional problems), and I'd do my best to show them movements and breathing techniques that could help, not just with the physical but with the emotional connection and connection to a bigger awareness. Plugging into the bigger awareness was always the "aha" moment for people. In truth the bigger awareness turns out to be everything. The aches and pains are symptoms of wear and tear that come from a disconnection from our inner power source. Once the pain is lifted, we are free once again, and we have the capacity to access our awareness. Physical pain became clear as a blocker of emotional happiness and freedom. Without our pain, we have nothing to cling to, and the expansive feeling of freedom can be frightening.

When I started playing around with guiding, I made it a quest to find ways to help people connect to themselves through physical movement. I did my best to get as clear as I could with simple language to help people move from here to there with ease. As I went further into my journey, I began leading classes in my apartment. Soon enough it became formal enough that my studio (aka apartment) needed a name. This is how Strala came to be.

Mike Taylor, my then boyfriend and now husband, who was also guiding people, and I sat on the floor and wrote down words we felt embodied the

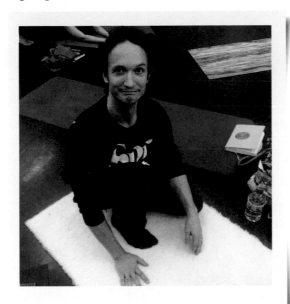

experience we had been aiming to deliver. We combined *strength*, *balance*, and *awareness* in a notebook and played around with the letters. *Strala* sounded like a great name. We liked the quality it held when you looked at the word and when you spoke it, so we went with it. As it turns out, the word means "to radiate light" in Swedish, which was pretty awesome synchronicity.

Strala has evolved over the years as a collaboration between Mike, Sam Berlind (a longtime shiatsu practitioner), and me. What started as a class I led in my apartment with a few friends once a day has grown naturally into a global movement with thousands of Guides, hundreds of thousands of regular practitioners,

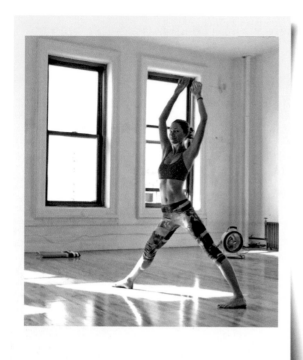

and, most exciting, a ripple in the fabric of modern yoga. Ease is the new/old way that has always led to great things. More people moving and living with ease is what is changing our world for the better.

This is my motivation for leading Strala. I want to help people enjoy sustainable well-being through practice of easygoing yoga and joyful living.

Now it's your turn. Ask yourself the simple, yet profound, question of why you want to guide. The answer will ground your work in authenticity and allow space for people to connect with you naturally.

Whatever your goals are, we live according to our intentions, whether we are aware or unaware of what they are. When our intentions are sustainable and full of love and service, we enjoy an endless supply of sustainable energy through the easy and challenging moments to do our work. When our intentions are for our own benefit, we become worn-out, tired, frustrated, and feel unsupported in our actions. It's a simple law of nature to do good things. Whether you choose to believe it or not on a philosophical level, your life has a much better chance of unfolding in your favor when you put your energy behind intentions of helping others than when you focus solely on helping yourself. Connecting with others is a fundamental part of who we are and is critical to our well-being.

Why do you want to (or currently) share yoga? The answer doesn't need to be profound, or completely formulated, but let it be specific and natural to you. There must be a story there of what led you to be here. It's probably emotional and full of passion. Maybe you experienced beneficial change or transformation through a regular practice of yoga and want to help others. Maybe yoga helped you recover from trauma. Maybe you came into yoga as a physical workout and ended up discovering the mind-body connection and got excited for more. No two stories are alike, and one of the most interesting ingredients that make you up as a Guide is the journey that brought you here. It's that journey, when you get real about it, that will ground you in the way you learn, communicate, and ultimately help people The more you get to know yourself and your intentions, the more you can help people in a great, sustainable way.

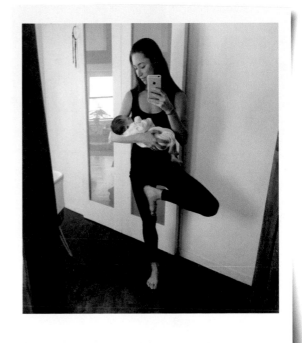

Once you are clear on your intention, you are ready to move into learning and embodying the key elements of Strala: the breath, the reminder to feel, and natural movement.

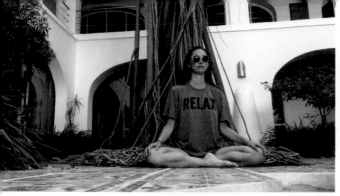
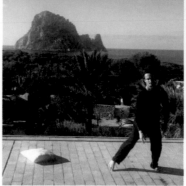

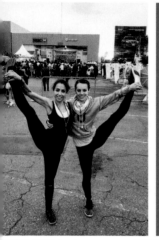

The fuller and deeper
you breathe, the more room
opens up inside.

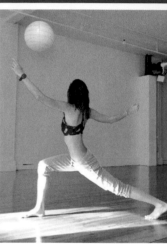

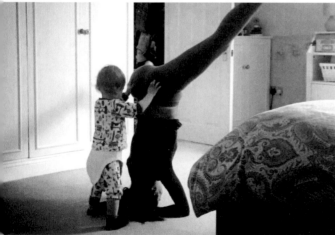
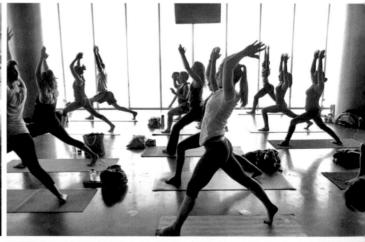

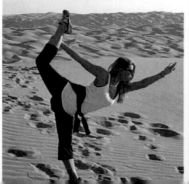
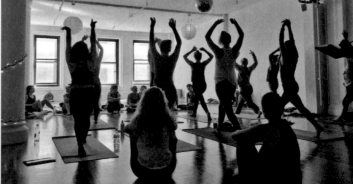

chapter
2

CREATE SPACE

THE BREATH-BODY CONNECTION

Imagine being in a vast, open space. The temperature is ideal. The sun shines. There is space around you to stretch out as much as you want. You feel open, calm, expansive, and free. You can run, jump, sit, or lie down and let your mind wander. We've all experienced something like this. Maybe it was in childhood, when the days felt long and endless. Maybe it was on a holiday where we were able to relax on a beach and enjoy the clouds as they passed by. Whatever the image that came to mind, I suspect you're feeling pretty happy because of it.

The great news is that it's possible to create more of these moments for ourselves and for those we lead. We can create this feeling in our lives, in our bodies, in the moments of our day-to-day life, in the here and now. This feeling of freedom and space is attainable with a radical yet completely natural approach to life and to practice. And it's all based on a renewable, inexhaustible resource we have with us all day long: the breath.

Our breath is the first building block to explore when looking at how we move in Strala Yoga. Breath is the basis for everything we do. Breathing deeply creates the space to move, explore, feel, and heal. There are two main uses of the breath in practice: to fuel our movement and to serve as a spotlight for feeling.

POWERING MOVEMENT & FINDING FEELING

Let's look at how the breath fuels movement. Try this. Sit easy wherever you are. Soften a bit. Take a big, huge, deep inhale. Exhale and relax.

Did you notice how your inhale actually moved your body for you? It helped you overcome that critical moment of inertia, when something not in motion gets set in motion. Once in motion, we, or any object, take less energy to stay in motion. Our options for movement are to move with or without the breath. We can simply lift our arm or leg, or we can soften, take a big inhale, and lift our arm or leg. The first option gets the job done, but we exhaust quickly. The second option allows the movement to become lighter, easier, and freer. By using the breath to fuel our movement, we can accomplish more with less effort, which leaves room to do more.

When we forget the breath, we can't achieve nearly as much because everything we do requires more effort. Inviting the breath to help move the body also allows space for us to feel and sensitize during the whole process. The benefits of using the breath are many, but that doesn't mean the choice to use it is easy. We have to decide that we will call on the power of ease and choose to believe that opening doors is better than breaking through them.

To use the breath to its fullest, we first need to soften. If we are stiff and tense, there is no room to breathe, no room to explore, and no ability to move.

the breath as fuel

STEP 1: Soften.

STEP 2: Breathe deeply.

STEP 3: Let your body go along for the ride.

First we soften. Then we breathe. The inhale moves us up, and the exhale takes us farther into a move. Try this. Take a big, deep inhale, and then a long, easy exhale. Let the breath move you. Let's try in a simple movement. Stand up tall with your feet apart enough so you can move easily. Soften here. There are two layers to softening: the mechanical and the emotional. Put a slight bend in your knees and elbows. This is your mechanical softening. To get the whole effect, we need to add the emotional softening. Allow your whole self to soften. If someone were to come over and give you a nudge, you would ripple like a wave but not fall over from your standing position. With the breath, we deal with our energy just as much as mechanics.

From your standing softening position, take a big inhale and float your arms up overhead. Exhale and soften your torso over your legs. Soften your knees and your whole self. Hang here for a few long, deep breaths, allowing your body to move how it feels good over your legs. When you're ready, roll yourself up to stand, take a big inhale, and float your arms up. Exhale and fold up and over your legs again. Hang here for a few long, deep breaths, and when you're ready, take your time and roll back up to standing. How did that go? Did you find more space open up in your body when you softened and let your breath move you? Did you feel longer and less rigid than usual?

Once we're comfortable with the idea of the breath as fuel for movement, we can begin to use it for its other purpose: to act as a spotlight for feeling. When we slow down enough to breathe deeply, we give ourselves space to explore what movement feels like in our body. We use the exploration to find a place that feels good. We use it to move past stress and tension. We step away from pain and settle into places that open the capacity to heal.

---

the breath as spotlight

STEP 1: Slow down.

STEP 2: Breathe deeply.

STEP 3: Explore and find.

As we create a breath-body connection and explore what feels good, we learn so much about ourselves. We find the excitement in us. We start to see what we are made of, and we become mesmerized. When we breathe into movement and explore, setting our attention inward, we see how at one with nature we are. Our ingredients are essentially stardust. It's a bummer we walk around forgetting how awesome and full of potential we are. Thankfully we can spend some time tapping in by using the breath. In fact, the breath is essential for our practice to come to life. Without it our movements are simply mechanical exercises. But with it we experience energy and spirit in our work, and we begin to see how truly magnificent we are.

THE MOVEMENT OF BREATH

Now let's move a little deeper into the practicalities. Using the breath changes the quality of our movements. They become soft, easygoing, and natural. Because of the breath, there are no end points. Just as an inhale shifts into an exhale without running into a corner or coming to a halt, the movements are easy and continuous when fueled by the breath.

The experience of moving with the breath is designed to feel oceanic. There is a calm ease carried through easy and challenging moments alike. The movements are designed to lift with each inhale and soften with each exhale, creating an expansive feeling physically and emotionally. The focus is on the process of the movement instead of the end point of a pose. This contributes to our ability to accomplish even difficult moves with ease. Our aim is to rest our focus and attention calmly on the breath, allowing space for a meditative experience.

In Strala we work in movement phrases guided by the concept of creating space by connecting the breath and the body. The inhale lifts, opens, and strengthens. The exhale moves farther, relaxes, and softens. The inhale does the work of moving the body: the breath lifts, and the body follows. The exhale does the job of moving you farther along in your pose: it rests you deeper into your movement.

There are a lot of cool ways to visualize this experience. On the inhale imagine a wave arcing. On the exhale the wave is rolling into shore. If we take this a step deeper, we can imagine the energy that is lifting and releasing the water. Our energy source is the breath—it lifts us and rolls us deeper into our experience. The breath is the energy, and the wave is our body. When we use the energy instead of muscling our way through movement, we become like a wave, deep, graceful, and powerful.

Using the breath enables us to move with ease. This isn't about being lazy; it's about being efficient. Obviously there is effort in any movement we do, but tapping into the power of the breath allows us to accomplish more with less effort. I know it's hard to let go of the force, push, struggle, and flexing of all the muscles, but it makes all the difference when you move through yoga and through the rest of life.

Using less energy allows you to do more. Using less energy allows you to rest your attention on your breath and access your creativity and intuition. Without the breath, you are wasting energy, and it's impossible to access those aha moments where your big ideas and answers to questions are resting. The reason things come to you when you are at rest is because you're not in the way of yourself, using up all your energy. Your mind has space to surprise you.

EXPERIENCE THE BREATH

The best way to see how powerful the breath can be is to experience it yourself. I'm going to take you through two exercises now so you can feel it in your own movements. First, I'll guide you through some movements frame by frame, but I won't give any specific directions about the breath. After you finish we'll take a look at how that felt, and then we'll move into the same movements again, this time with breath guidance included.

MOVING WITHOUT THE BREATH

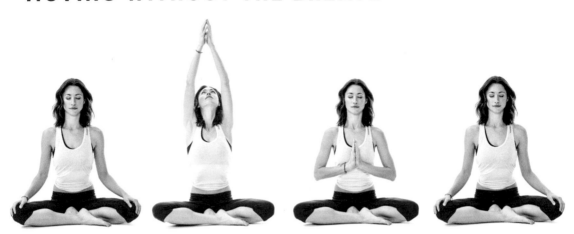

Sit comfortably. Lift your arms up. Press your palms together. Bring your thumbs to your heartbeat. Inhale through your nose. Exhale through your mouth. Twice more like that. Inhale through your nose. Exhale through your mouth. Inhale through your nose. Exhale through your mouth. Relax your hands on your thighs.

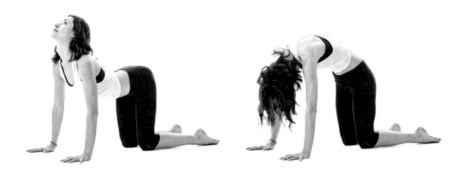

Come onto all fours. Drop your belly, arch your back, and look up. Round your back and look down. Repeat this three times.

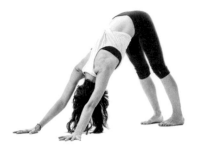

Tuck your toes and lift your hips up and back to down dog.

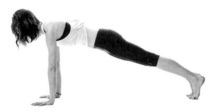

Tuck your chin and roll out to plank. Hold here for a few seconds.

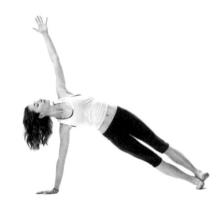

Shift your weight onto your right hand and the outside edge of your right foot, and open your body to your left. Hold here for a few seconds. Come back to plank and move to the other side. Come back to plank.

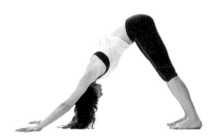

Lift your hips and press back to down dog.

Lift your right leg up behind you. Open your hips.

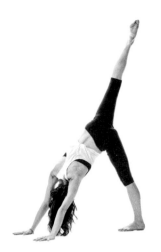

Step your right foot through to low lunge. Come onto your fingertips and sink your hips low.

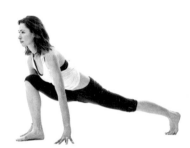

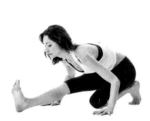

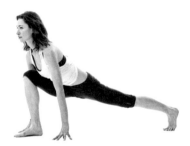

Lower your back knee to the ground and sink your hips to your back heel. Relax your torso over your front leg. Hold here for a few seconds. Crawl yourself back to low lunge.

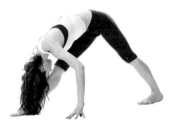

Press your fingertips on the ground, lift your hips up, and relax your torso over your front leg. Hold here for a few seconds. Sink your hips back to low lunge.

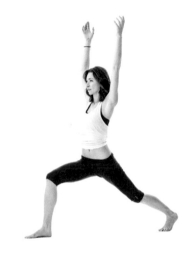

Press down through your legs and lift up into high lunge, lifting your hips up and arms up overhead.

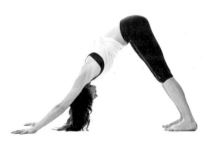

Come back into low lunge, plant your palms, and step back to down dog.

REFLECTION MOMENT: How did that feel? Ask yourself how you feel, first intellectualizing what happened in the movement phrase. Begin to deconstruct how to create an ideal feeling and experience. When we work with how we feel, we get to the root of how we'd like to shift the experience. From there we can look at language, tone, body position, and all the ingredients that factor into the experience.

So grab your journal and write down how you feel. Express yourself in words, phrases, or sentences, however you see fit. Below is some of the feedback other Guides from around the world provided when they did this exercise.

❋ The movement felt fine but uninspired.

❋ I found myself thinking, *Am I doing this right, or when will it be finished?*

❋ I felt myself stopping and starting a lot.

❋ I felt like I was being told what to do.

❋ I felt unbalanced and a little stiff.

❋ I felt like I was going too fast or not fast enough.

❋ It was okay, but just movement, without any mind-body or emotional connection.

❋ The experience felt tense and rigid.

How does your feedback match up? It's amazing the problems that arise with the absence of the breath. Suddenly a simple sequence feels unbalanced and stiff. Absent breath cues, the Guide appears very "in charge" in a "do what I tell you right now and you have no choice" kind of way. The experience of connecting to the self and the freedom that brings is replaced with the requirement to please someone outside yourself. Minds frazzle, intuition is squashed, and the ease vanishes. Our breath is the magical force that carries us. Our breath is the gateway that makes feeling possible. With the breath gone, we are limited to static, flat, labored positioning.

Let's go again, this time with the full, deep breath.

MOVING WITH THE BREATH

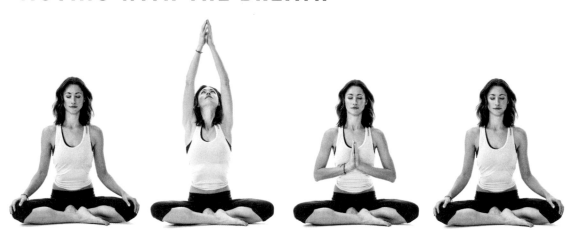

Sit comfortably. Take a big inhale and lift your arms up. Press your palms together. Bring your thumbs to your heartbeat. Soften here for a moment. Take a big inhale through your nose. Long exhale through your mouth. Twice more like that. Big inhale through your nose. Long exhale through your mouth. Big inhale through your nose. Long exhale through your mouth. Relax your hands on your thighs.

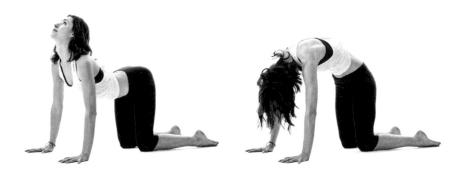

Come onto all fours easy with your breath. Take a big inhale, dropping your belly, arching your back, and looking up. Exhale and round your back and look down. Roll around here how it feels good to you, letting your breath lead your movements.

When you're ready, tuck your toes, take a big inhale, and lift your hips up and back to down dog. Soften here for a few breaths. Sway a bit side to side if that feels nice to you.

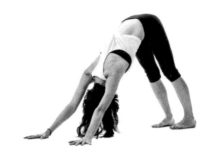

Tuck your chin and roll out to plank. Soften here for a few moments. Sway a bit side to side and forward and back if that feels nice.

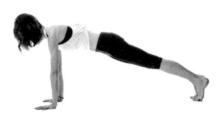

Shift your weight onto your right hand and the outside edge of your right foot, take a big inhale, and open your body to your left. Hang here for a few moments, opening up. Come back to plank, take a big inhale, and open up to your other side. Hang here for a few moments. Come back to plank.

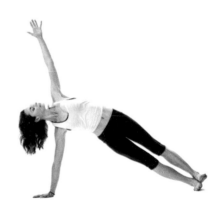

Take a big inhale and lift your hips up and back to down dog. Soften here for a moment.

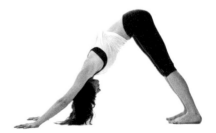

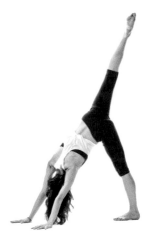

Take a big inhale and lift your right leg up behind you. Open your hips if that feels nice.

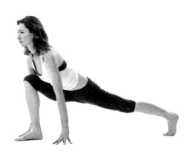

Step your right foot through to low lunge. Come onto your fingertips and sink your hips low. Sway around here if that feels good.

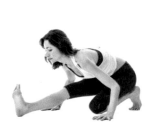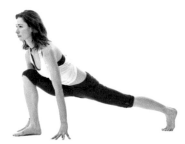

Soften your back knee to the ground and sink your hips toward your back heel. Relax your torso over your front leg. Hang here for a few moments breathing really full and deep. Crawl yourself back to low lunge.

Press your fingertips on the ground, take a big inhale, lift your hips up, and relax your torso over your front leg. Hang here for a few seconds. Sway a bit side to side if that feels nice. Sink your hips back to low lunge.

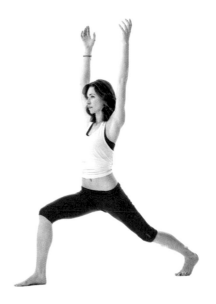

Press down through your legs, take a big inhale, and lift up to high lunge, lifting your hips up and your arms up overhead.

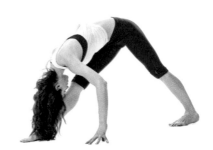

Exhale and soften back into low lunge, plant your palms, and make your way back to down dog.

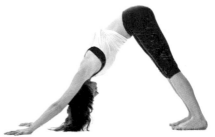

REFLECTION MOMENT: How did *that* feel? Grab your journal and write it down. Notice how you felt during and after the movements.

I haven't met anyone yet who didn't prefer to be guided with the breath. Even experienced yogis who talk about knowing when to breathe in and out appreciate the support of the verbal cuing. It feels like encouragement and has a beautiful way of zapping rigidity and tension out of the room. Here is a list of the most universal feedback for this experience.

✳ It was easier with the breath.

✳ I felt supported.

✳ I could do more with less effort.

✳ I felt like I had all the time I wanted.

✳ It went by so fast.

✳ I know the movements were challenging, but they felt easy with the breath.

✳ I felt lighter in my body.

✳ I felt connected to how I feel.

✳ I felt like I was in charge of my practice and had a nice support.

It's incredible how big a difference guiding the breath makes. Of course, if no one is guiding you, you will still be breathing, but you won't be using the breath for the fuel that it is. Movements that are easy become difficult and disjointed. Movements that are challenging become impossible. The general vibe is stressed, worried, and competitive.

The breath-body connection opens up everything, from allowing challenges to become easier, relaxation to become deeper and more healing, and strength building to become safer and more efficient to space for the experience to feel simply amazing.

As you go through your practice, I encourage you to pay attention to the breath. Are there moments when you notice you aren't breathing? If so, how do you feel when it happens? Try shifting your focus from breathing and moving to breathing fully and deeply and allowing your whole self to go along for the ride. An amazing shift is possible. The breath does the work, and you begin to ride the meditative wave of your own powerful inhale and exhale—and all the moments in between.

Make room for you. Take a big, deep inhale. Long, easy exhale. Enjoy!

The path you take
to get where you're going
will affect how you feel
once you get there.

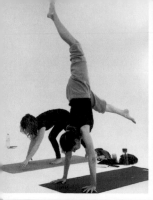
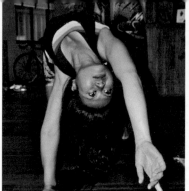
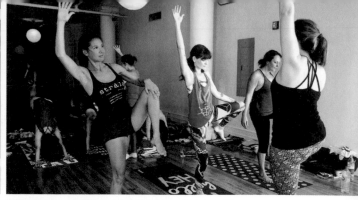

The path you take to get where you're going will affect how you feel once you get there.

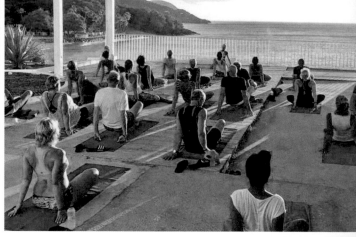

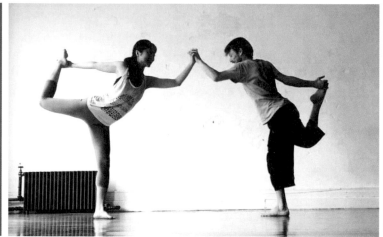

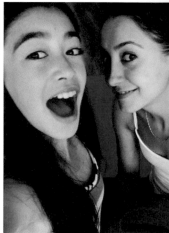

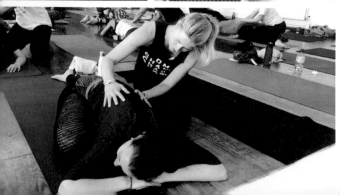

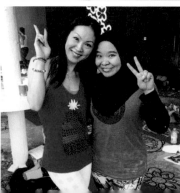

FOLLOW YOUR INTUITION

A REMINDER TO FEEL

The next element in Strala movement that we need to explore is feeling. We discussed this a little in Chapter 2, in terms of using the breath to shine a spotlight on feeling, but let's go a bit deeper.

This concept of tapping into how you feel is foreign to so many of us. We've been pushed and prodded to work through the pain, tightness, and discomfort. We've practiced this so much that we've lost our ability to feel. We're so used to cutting ourselves off from feeling that our bodies have stopped communicating with us, and we have no idea if we feel good or bad. But feeling is essential if you want to move in ways that will lead to enhanced energy, creativity, and healing.

Why is this? We are different from day to day, from morning to night, from month to month, from year to year, and from one side of the body to the other side. When we feel in our practice, we don't look the same each time. And that's good. We're going for an internal experience that allows us to sustainably accomplish more with less effort. Our goal is to feel good in the process, not to reach a certain shape or pose. By moving in this way, we take away the pressure of competition—with ourselves and with others. The focus moves to your moment-to-moment experience rather than an end goal.

Sensitizing to how we feel is the real prize of practice. It leads to a deeper connection to your intuition and creativity, and it allows space for physical and emotional healing. When we focus on feeling in our movements, we get in the flow of how our body moves best, which helps us easily build strength and a healthy range of mobility. Moving this way also allows the relaxation response to ignite, bodies to heal, and minds to clear.

We also simply enjoy the process more. If we are used to checking off a to-do list every day, following a set of rules to get things done with the goal of achieving something, at best we might end up achieving that goal, but we will have beaten ourselves up the whole way. Ironically, working in this way often makes us not even enjoy reaching that goal. By not feeling, we miss out on exploration during the process, and exploration is what lets us enjoy the journey.

We also open possibilities to move and achieve beyond our set goal when we pay attention to how we feel and explore. When we move with feeling, we move only in ways that feel good. This conserves energy, and because we're not taxing ourselves, we allow room to do more work. Our vision of possibilities widens when we participate in the process instead of checking off items on a list. With feeling we replace rigidity and frustration with grace and ease and take ourselves to fantastic places every step of the way.

On the other end of the spectrum, when we shut off feeling, we get into trouble in yoga and loads of other circumstances. Have you ever been in a situation that was challenging and responded by shutting down, clenching up, and sort of just waiting for it to be over? I think it's safe to say that we all have a version of this reaction in our personal history. Our practice is a wonderful place to work on how we are under any circumstance, while we are dealing with ourselves, so we can have a more effective time of it with the rest of our lives. When we practice following how we feel on the mat, we become masters of ease off the mat, as well.

GETTING SENSITIZED

Getting into feeling mode is the practice of paying attention to how you feel and responding accordingly. It requires all the practices we have discussed so far: slowing down, breathing deeply, and exploring. There is no one correct destination when it comes to feeling. It is simply a mindful exploration of yourself while moving slowly and easily enough to find your way into some great places. In essence, it's the experience of in-motion self-awareness.

Exploration is the essence of getting sensitized, but exploration is not something that is encouraged in life. While it was once an inherent part of our being—as seen in a child's curiosity and play—exploration becomes devalued as we grow up. Society teaches us to stuff this desire deep down into ourselves so we can focus on doing what we're "supposed" to do. We set aside exploration for a time of planned slacking off—a time when we don't have to follow the rules. But exploration shouldn't be seen as slacking off. It is in our nature. Without it we walk blindly through our lives, simply following the programming set by other people, which makes us no different from a washing machine. Fortunately, we are composed of elements that thrive on connection to the self and our surroundings, so tapping into this feels rewarding immediately. We derive immense value from softening, breathing deeply, slowing down, and feeling so we can respond properly to what we need in the moment. Responding is the action that comes from feeling—and responding is what we can practice.

To practice responding to how we feel, we must be tuned in enough to realize that we have a choice. And then we choose what's best for us. In the context of a yoga practice, this means we notice we feel a little jammed up in the hips, so we back off, slow down, and explore around the pose, instead of pushing our bodies farther into one position. We gently move a little left or right or around, searching for ease. In our exploration we shine a light on the path to the most useful places to spend time, and in these places we spend a few moments, breathing deeply, to give proper care to our tight hips. If we forget feeling, we stay in the pose and do our best to make our bodies open up with force. But using force against resistance is a recipe for more tension and injury. When you go to war with yourself, someone is going to lose, and that someone is always you. It's much better if you win, and without a struggle is even nicer.

getting sensitized

Tune in.

Respond.

Believe what you experience.

Slow down.

Breathe deeply.

Explore.

When we use feeling as our guide, the cues about what to do come from within. The experience moves from external to internal. The benefits shift from minimal to maximal: you get an improved, healthy range of mobility; sensitization toward what's going on with your body; and connection to your emotional, mental, and physical state of being. Yoga has been disguised by poses for many years. It's our job as practitioners to bring ourselves and those around us back to feeling, so we can navigate to some amazing places. All the great, cool yoga magic happens when we are connected to feeling and respond accordingly.

THE STRUGGLE OF SELF-AWARENESS

One of the biggest issues people have with tapping into feeling is that they've been trained to not feel. I know I've mentioned this before, but it's one of the hardest challenges to overcome as you work your way into the Strala philosophy. Many of us have spent so much time cutting ourselves off from feeling that starting to feel leaves us riddled with doubt. We doubt that the path of ease can take us far toward health and well-being. We doubt what our bodies are telling us. We doubt all the information that goes against what we've been programmed to believe. The struggle is real, and it can be very hard to allow ourselves to feel. It can be scary. But it's worth it. To rekindle our lines of communication with our bodies, we simply need to practice. Tune in again and again. Choose to believe the information we're getting. Respond accordingly and watch the results. It takes a lot of time to reprogram the belief that we need to push through and accomplish, accomplish, accomplish. But it's possible—and so rewarding.

Moving from force to ease was truly a struggle for me. Growing up, I was so focused on doing good and accomplishing what I had my heart set on that I looked at feeling as a sign of weakness. "What am I doing?" and "How will I get there?" were the constant questions in my head. "How am I feeling?" was irrelevant. To ask myself about my feelings or if I was living in accordance with them seemed like an unnecessary waste of time—or worse, laziness. As I've grown up a bit, I've realized that, in so many ways, I was missing the point of what I was doing. Feeling is the center of all things amazing. Without feeling goals may be accomplished, but they have less intrinsic value and less meaning. Without feeling we lack connection to ourselves and the world around us. Without feeling our actions are based around fear. Once I realized this, I became properly obsessed with feeling. Not simply feeling good but exploring how I felt for the sake of purpose and direction. This isn't an exercise in hedonism; it's an exercise in being alive, fully present, aware, and electrically you—both on and off the mat.

There is no perfect way to master feeling; it's a lifelong, highly rewarding process if you're brave enough to step out of your comfort zone and slow down, soften, and listen to the conversation inside. The path you take to get where you're going will affect how you feel once you're there.

OPPORTUNITIES TO EXPLORE

Now that you understand the basics of feeling, let's drill down a little into one element: opportunities to explore. There are moments in many phrases when we're in a position or around a position for more than one deep inhale or exhale. This variety gives depth and rhythm to your phrases and waves. If you watch the ocean for a while, you'll notice all the waves are different. You can spend hours getting drawn into their subtle changes in height, volume, and quality. Phrases can be as captivating and visceral as an afternoon with the ocean when you let your whole being get involved in the experience.

In most places in the class, the movement, initiated with the breath, flows continuously from one moment to the next. But in some places in the movement phrases, there are moments where you have an opportunity to linger for a capsulated experience. For example, it makes sense to linger in pigeon pose and take several long, deep breaths. During this time you can explore the pose and find a great place to settle. Even when you are seemingly still, your breath is subtly lifting and softening you along. As you feel what happens during this capsulated experience, you sensitize yourself to have an internal versus external experience. This changes the practice from static poses to a conversation with yourself.

EXPERIENCE FEELING

Let's experience how important feeling is in the practice to see how much of a difference it makes. I'm going to take you through two exercises now so you can feel it in your own movements. First, I'll guide you through some movements, but I won't give any specific directions about feeling. After you finish we'll take a look at how that felt, and then we'll move into the same movements again, this time with feeling guidance included.

GUIDING WITHOUT FEELING

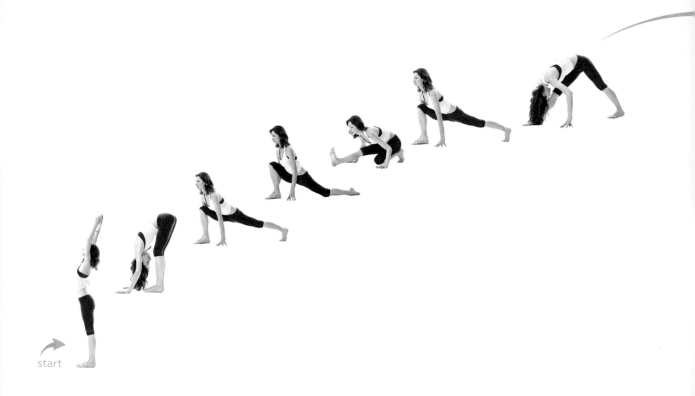

start

Start standing, soften your knees a bit here. Take a big inhale and lift your arms up. Exhale and soften over your legs into a forward bend. Soften your knees, press your fingertips on the ground, and step your left leg back to a low lunge. Ease your back knee down. Now bring your hips back toward your back heel for your runner's stretch. Relax your torso over your front leg. Now crawl yourself back out to your low lunge. Press your fingertips down, lift your hips up, and fold your torso over your front leg. Now press down through your legs, take a big inhale, and lift up into a high lunge. Ground your back heel down and soften into warrior 2. Take a big inhale and lift your hips and arms up. Exhale and soften back into warrior 2. Take a big

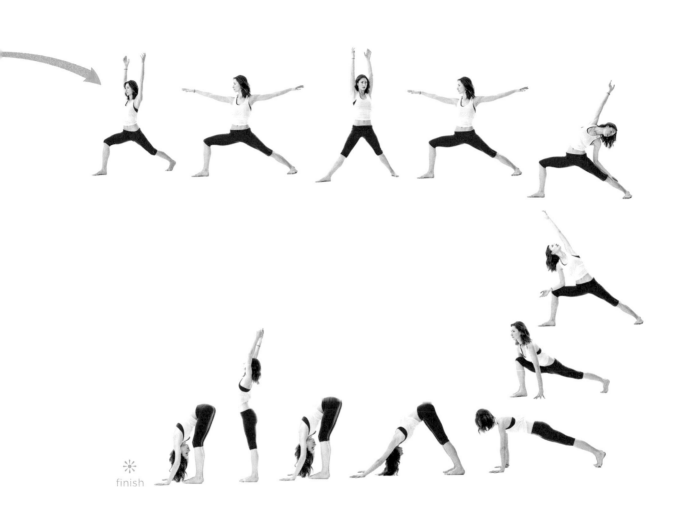

✳
finish

inhale and tip back to reverse warrior. Bring yourself up and over, pressing your right forearm on your thigh and opening your left arm up and overhead and rolling your belly open. Now bring your fingertips to the ground on either side of your front foot coming into low lunge. Plant your palms on the ground and step back to plank. Take a big inhale and lift your hips up and back to down dog. Take an easy stroll up to the top of your mat one step at a time. Relax your torso over your legs. Round up to stand one notch at a time. Take a big inhale and lift your arms up. Exhale and soften back over your legs. Repeat the whole phrase on your other side.

REFLECTION MOMENT: How did that feel? Chances are it wasn't too horrible, but we can do much better. There is a feeling of space missing. Empowerment and self-awareness go missing. Without the feeling reminders the Guide first becomes desensitized so no matter what words are said, it's impossible to give feeling to others. So we've lost the example, and we've lost the sense of time and space that feeling gives. The breath cues, although they are present, are less effective. We can do better. I want you to feel better.

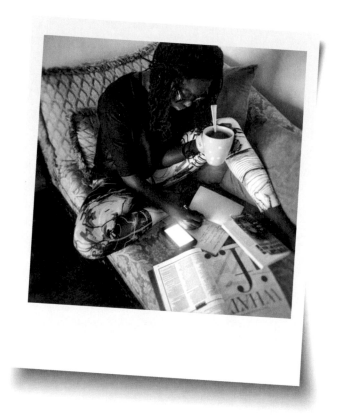

So grab your journal and write down how you feel. Express yourself in words, phrases, or sentences, however you see fit. Below is some of the feedback other Guides from around the world have provided when they did this exercise.

＊ I felt like the teacher was ordering me around, and I was not in charge of my body.

＊ I felt always late or early into the next movement, but never on time.

＊ Those movements are usually easy for me, and now they were suddenly hard.

＊ I felt like I was being bossed around.

＊ The environment felt stiff.

＊ I felt like I was in trouble.

＊ It was okay, but just movement, without any mind-body or emotional connection.

How does your feedback match up? It's amazing the problems that arise with the absence of feeling. It's scary what we are used to in our lives, as well. Without the feeling cues, all the lovely work we've done with the breath is essentially useless. Leading is about matching how you are with what you say in a clear and effective way. You need both to match up, and that is part of the quest of improving. It's not an easy thing to pick up and master, but it's a worthy endeavor and I know you can be a great Guide helping people reconnect with themselves. It's who you naturally are.

Let's go again, this time with the full, deep breath and the feeling.

MOVING WITH THE BREATH & FEELING

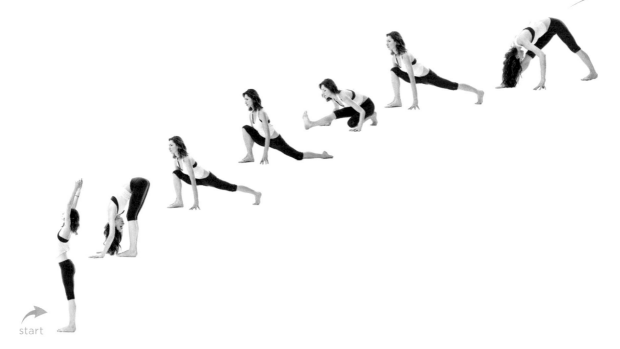

start

Start standing easy, soften your knees a bit here. Take a big inhale and lift your arms up. Exhale and soften over your legs into a forward bend. Soften your knees, press your fingertips on the ground, and step your left leg back to a low lunge. Ease your back knee down. If it feels nice to hang your torso low, go for that. If it feels nicer to open up your torso, go for that, breathing really big and full and deep. When you're ready, bring your hips back toward your back heel for your runner's stretch. Relax your torso over your front leg. Sway a bit side to side if that feels nice. When you're ready, crawl yourself back out to your low lunge. Press your fingertips down, lift your hips up, and fold your torso over your front leg. Sway a bit side to side if that feels nice. When you're ready, press down through your legs, take a big inhale, and lift up into a high lunge. Ground your back heel down and soften into warrior 2. Take a big inhale and lift your hips and arms up. Exhale and soften back into warrior 2. Take a big inhale and tip back to reverse warrior. Bring yourself up and over, pressing your right forearm on your thigh and opening your left arm up and overhead and rolling your belly open. Bring your fingertips to the ground on either side of your front foot coming into low lunge. Plant your palms on the ground and step back to plank. Take a big inhale and lift your hips up and back to down dog. Take an easy stroll up to the top of your mat

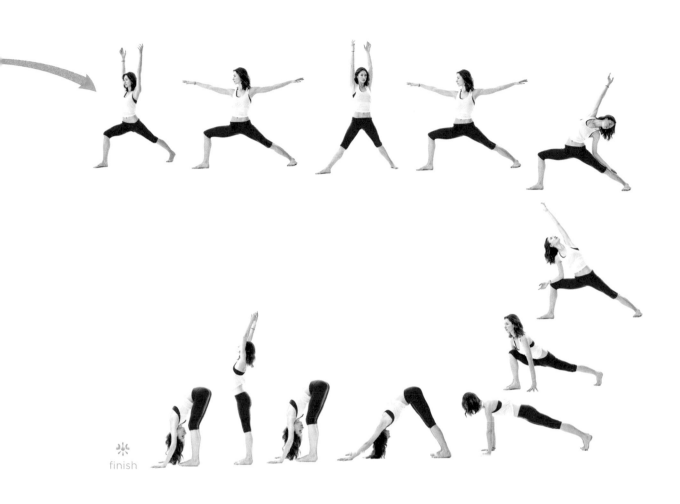

finish

one step at a time. Once you make it up, relax your torso over your legs. Round up to stand one notch at a time. Take a big inhale and lift your arms up. Exhale and soften back over your legs. Repeat the whole phrase on your other side.

REFLECTION MOMENT: How did that feel? Take out your journal and write if you feel inspired. The amazing thing about the potential of yoga is that it reminds us that we are nature. Nature is a powerful example of feeling and individuality existing together. The trees all sway in the breeze, but they don't do it exactly the same way. The tree sways exactly the way the tree needs to sway, and each tree does that, providing a wonderfully unique and cohesive forest. Your yoga class can be this wonderful and gorgeous when you clearly lead from how you are and what you say breath and feeling together. Otherwise we might as well be doing synchronized aerobics.

The breath-body cues open the space to feel. The breath lifts, and the body follows. Do you see how important it is to slow down, soften, and breathe deeply? Do you see how doing this leads you right to feeling? There is no need for me to tell you, "Just feel" or "Let it go" or some other flowery-feeling cue.

If we were to take these reminder cues out, the experience shifts. The feeling cues provide a clear and safe path for you to move in a way that feels great for you. Most people feel that these cues let them move in their own time, while simultaneously being part of the group experience. Any pressure to do certain poses or to be in a competition dissolves.

UNEXPECTED CAPSULES OF EXPLORATION

Opportunities to explore present themselves all over our classes. They aren't just in the obvious places like pigeon pose, seated forward bend, and final relaxation. They can surprise us in places like single leg forward bend, twisted half moon, down dog, and handstand. Our continuous phrases allow feeling through graceful movement. Our opportunities to explore allow feeling through slowing down, softening, and deciding where and how to move within the phrase. Any moment where you are allowed some space to linger is an opportunity to explore.

Let's look at the process of doing a handstand, which provides us with some unexpected opportunities to explore. The movements leading up to and following the handstand—and the handstand itself—provide a few moments of open space to explore.

In the spirit of honoring our inner sixth grade sentence diagramming, we'll explore the complete handstand sentence—starting with standing split and ending with down dog. I'll let you decide what pieces should be the nouns, verbs, and adjectives. It's all action and waves to me.

The visual below shows us a way of organizing what we're about to do. It shows what's happening, other things that could happen at the same time, and where we are going to meet up.

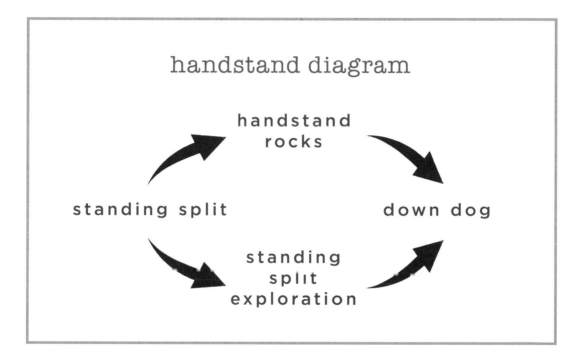

It's like walking to a planned destination with a friend. You could walk up the same street you always take, or you could choose to walk around another way. Either way, they are both lovely walks, you're in good company, and you're headed toward your destination together.

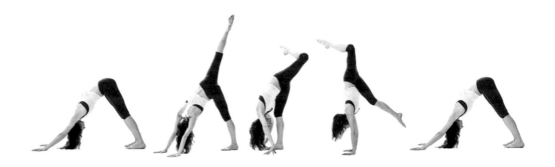

So let's start with a down dog. Spread your fingers like you're digging into wet sand. Soften your knees and elbows a bit and sway side to side if that feels nice. Walk your feet toward your hands, leaving a couple feet between your hands and feet. Take a big inhale and lift your right leg up to down dog split. Open your hips and shoulders here. Exhale and soften your knees a bit and roll around in your hips. Plant your palms on the ground and rock forward and back, moving from your hips. Inhale to rock forward, bringing your hips over your shoulders. Exhale, soften back. Roll through this a few times if you'd like, or explore here in your standing split. Eventually we'll meet up in down dog. When you're ready go for the other side.

REFLECTION MOMENT: How did that feel? Were you able to bring a bit of exploration into your handstand? Take some notes in your journal about this experience. Perhaps you noticed that by saying, "Eventually we'll meet up in down dog," I created a capsulated moment for freedom and exploration. This is a wonderful way to practice a handstand. It gives you a clear process, with an option to explore—either in handstand or in the easier standing split. Ultimately this exploration leads to a handstand without force. It is a prime example of focusing on the process yet blowing past the goal.

THREE STEPS TO FEELING

To sum up the practice of tapping into feeling, I want to turn to Mike Taylor here. When he talks about feeling, he lays out a nice, three-step process that a lot of people find really helpful. So let's turn it over to him. Take a big, full, deep breath and enjoy!

MIKE:

Imagine for a moment that you go to yoga to do poses. Of course that's not why you started all this. But you get to the yoga room, and that's what the teacher is explaining to you, in great detail. Poses. There's even a lot of talk about your bones, and where to put them. So there you are, posing and thinking about what to do with your bones.

At best you'll probably get bored fast. The teacher has you thinking, rather than feeling. If the teacher wants me to get stuck in my head, I'd really rather not think about my bones. I'd rather think about pancakes. So there I am thinking about pancakes. Now we're here because it's supposed to be good for us, and we're waiting for it to be over. Because the pancakes, or whatever we're thinking about, aren't here.

So that's at best: bored and tuned out from how you feel. But at worst you're aiming for poses and struggling to do them right. This inevitably puts more stress and strain into your body and mind. So you'll inject your body full of cortisol, and you'll feel sore and tense from your yoga. You'll be open to frequent injury, hypermobility in your joints, and chronic pain.

Imagine now that you're here to feel. Really feel. In an instant, every inch that you move through becomes completely fascinating. Getting to know you becomes completely fascinating. You inspire yourself. Stress and tension dissolve. Your body fills with oxytocin. You're connected, tuned in. You become your own best caregiver. You get radiantly healthy. You get happy. And it's never over. You carry this feeling, this ability to connect, in everything you do. Why wouldn't you? It feels indescribably amazing.

Want to create this shift in your yoga? Want to share this with everyone around you? Of course!

Strala creates this wonderful shift in yoga, from what is too often a stress inducing experience of poses, to a meditative experience of yourself.

It's not about memorizing external rules, faithfully copied from a guru who has never seen you. It's not about experiencing poses. It's not even about yoga.

It's about you, experiencing you.

How does this work? There are three major parts to creating your own shift. From here, you'll have something wonderful to share.

1. SHIFT IN FOCUS: FROM RULES TO FEELING. For many decades, yoga has focused on what the poses look like. Rules of alignment are rigidly applied, trying to fit everyone into the same correct shape. Of course, this doesn't make much sense. We're all unique. We have our own backgrounds and health histories. Your shape isn't my shape or her shape, and that's a good thing! We become the best version of ourselves when we aim to create the best version of ourselves, not a version of someone else.

Strala moves the focus from an external rules-driven experience of poses, to an internal experience of yourself. How you feel is the guide, not a picture, not rules invented by someone else, for someone else. Strala creates a structure for connecting with yourself, and becoming extremely capable at working with what you've got.

2. SHIFT IN GOALS: FROM END POINTS TO NOW. Most yoga philosophy would agree that poses aren't so important. What is in your mind is. The direct experience of yourself is. But when yoga practice begins, philosophy flies out the window. Instruction is all about getting into and perfecting the poses.

Strala brings yoga philosophy and practice together as the same thing. The poses aren't the goal. It's not more vital to be in one particular position—a pose—than any other position. Every inch of you is equally crucial. Every inch you can move through is equally important. So the pose isn't the goal. Feeling good is the goal. You are the goal.

By dropping the linear pose goals, the end points, Strala brings you into the direct experience of exactly where you are, now. You're not aiming for poses. You're no longer aiming to be somewhere you are not. You're just here to feel and get to know you.

So what about the poses? Remarkably, getting to know your body and mind in this non-goal-oriented way makes the poses just not that hard anymore. When you know yourself, and have the experience of working easily with everything you've got, difficult things become easy.

3. SHIFT IN SOURCE: FROM OUTSIDE TO INSIDE. Have you learned the correct way to ground your hands and feet, rotate your shoulders and thighs, suck in your belly, and fix your gaze? Forget it. All of it.

If you want to do easy things the hard way, these rules are all useful. I've seen generations of yoga teachers make a big, intimidating fuss about the simplest things in this way. It's likely in the guru handbook, how to keep your followers following you! But there's another way.

If you'd like to do hard things the easy way, that doesn't come from rules. It comes from you, knowing you. It won't look like what anyone has ever done before. It will look like you. It will look like how you feel.

Strala shifts the source from external to internal. The teacher, the rules of alignment, shapes, and studies are not the source of knowledge. *You* are the source. Yoga can become an external experience of other people's rules, applied to my body, adopted from gurus who have never seen me. Yoga can also become an internal experience of yourself. No rigid rules, no correct ways, just what you find each day.

It's empowering that you are the source. Since it's self-creating, rather than receiving and copying, it also takes effort. But most important, it's probably the only way that really works, for each of us. It might not apply so well to flying a plane. Or open-heart surgery. But it applies well to your yoga. And it applies very well to your health and your life.

Strala isn't a system to control people. It's a system to free people. That's why Strala feels so good. It's probably also why Strala people accomplish with such inspiring ease what is considered so challenging. It's not about yoga. It's about you.

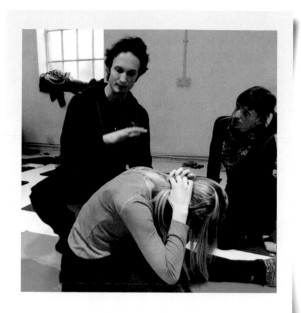

BE YOUR FIRST RESPONDER

Becoming sensitized to how you feel and comfortable believing and responding to what you feel are tremendously valuable skills to develop. If you go through life ignoring how you feel until your body stops communicating with you, you will eventually lose. Buckets full of stress, sickness, and disease creep in. Hopefully you'll receive a wake-up call and get back on the bandwagon of listening and self-care before it's too late. Prevention is the best cure, and there is a lot we can do to take good care of ourselves through listening and responding. We can start on the mat and enjoy the effect in the rest of our lives. I know firsthand that I used to catch a cold every season. I would get tired and stressed, have problems sleeping, and feel disconnected. With a regular practice of following how I feel, I now rarely get sick—with anything, let alone a cold. I can also manage stress better, sleep like a baby, and feel generally positive, energetic, and happy. When I started listening to how I feel, my life shifted pretty dramatically, and I'm grateful for this every day. You have the power to feel like this too. Remember, it's not the yoga that heals you; it's you that heals you.

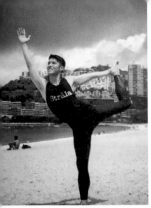
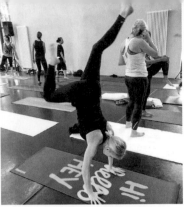
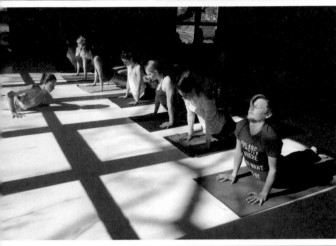
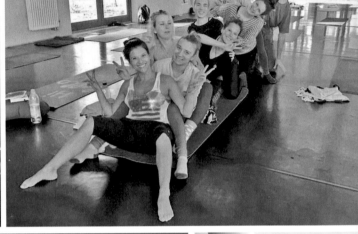
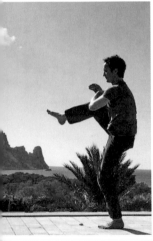

"

Move in agreement with yourself
and you'll be in the flow
of all the magic.

"

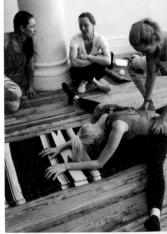
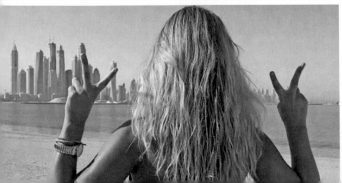
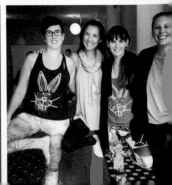

chapter

4

FLOW LIKE WATER

FINDING NATURAL MOVEMENT

The final piece of the Strala philosophy is natural movement.
This is the action of doing the most possible with the least amount of effort. It's
the how of getting around in your body during the practice.

    With natural movement we move softly and consistently, from the middle.
Leading from the hips and belly, we stay on balance, wherever we go. There are
no end points. We don't stop and start. We don't immobilize our bodies in an
effort to hold a pose. We simply move in ways that feel good. This is a radical
suggestion in a yoga practice, but it's oh so normal in nature. Water flows. Wind
blows. Even when we can't see any outward sign of movement, the current softly
rises and settles.

We soften before we move, soften before we lift, soften before we roll. It's amazing that so much power comes from the action of softening. Natural movement contributes greatly to building strength, healthy mobility, and safety. The movement comes from the inside out. The body is soft as it moves. There is no need to clench and flex the muscles. As soon as we clench, we immobilize ourselves and introduce agitation. When we relax and move softly, from the inside out, with no end points, our capabilities are limited only by our imaginations.

SAFETY & MOVEMENT

Because of its focus on natural movement, Strala is safe for everyone—every age, every size, every injury history, and every health background. If there's a pose we don't do, it means this pose isn't particularly good for some people. Our approach creates a healthy balance between strength and flexibility, stability and mobility. This is why we don't jump, push, or aim for hypermobility in poses that put strain on vulnerable areas like the spine, shoulders, wrists, hips, and knees. These are all common areas for yoga injuries, and these injuries don't happen with Strala. We just heal them.

Once you become a highly experienced yoga practitioner, you can do the hard poses in a way that encompasses the idea of natural movement. You will know your body so well, through sensitizing yourself to how you feel and finding the best-feeling ways to do everything, that you will be able to handle almost any pose and feel really good while doing it.

So keep moving easy, everything you've got, in every direction you can move it. If something hurts, if something immobilizes you with tension, don't do it. Back off just enough that you're easily and happily movable again. Explore in every direction from here, and your comfort zone will gradually expand. Eventually the things that were hard just won't be hard anymore, and you'll get there without stress or injury.

11 PRINCIPLES OF NATURAL MOVEMENT

Mike Taylor is not only my husband; he's also an agent of ease. Mike was brought up with a no-rules philosophy to movement and accomplished a lot in athletics with this completely different approach. When he was a teen and in his early 20s, he won a ton of martial arts competitions in Asia, the kind they don't talk about, and it took me almost six years to get the full story—I think I have it now. Because of his training, Mike can do loads of ninja stuff with his body, and he does it all with ease. It's all so natural that it looks simple—even when he's doing the hardest move you can find. That's why I felt like he would be the best one to tell you all about the 11 principles of natural movement. Let him be your guide into moving easily, with everything you've got, in every direction:

Pose-based yoga has become increasingly common lately—even among professional athletes. On the surface, I understand why this is. There are some benefits. For example, holding poses can have a pacifying effect on some people, which might help to quiet down a super-loud mind. Also the unusual shapes we take in yoga get us into parts of our body we don't usually discover, and it's useful to discover everything we have. Pose-based yoga can also help us learn that we can do more than we believed possible. So these are good things.

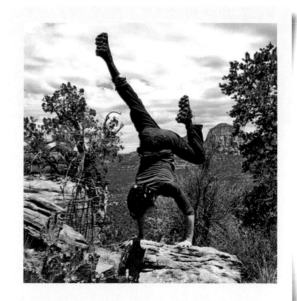

But pose-based yoga also leads to increased incidence of strains, sprains, and tendinitis and bursitis in tendons, ligaments, muscles, and joints. Trying to fit yourself into a specific pose introduces tension into your body. And when a body is tense, it resists easy movement. However, because of the focus of the pose, we push past the resistance to get to a specific shape. By forcing our bodies to do things they don't want to, we hurt ourselves. These injuries often require extended healing time, which is bad for the average person and terrible for a professional athlete.

But I think we can learn a lot from a professional athlete when we watch them take part in the sport at which they excel. When we see them in the flow of play, we see that they have everything: mobility and agility, power and endurance. They move smoothly, using only the energy they need to make that basket, pass that ball, or balance through that kick. In short, a great athlete is never working against himself or herself. Which really is a nice way to be for all of us.

The key here, for all of us, is to move like pro athletes do when they're moving at their prime. They are moving as their bodies tell them to. They are moving naturally. We all need to return to natural movement. I say "return" because so often, nature—even our own nature—becomes unnatural to us. We are so used to tuning out and ignoring how we feel that we disconnect from the direct feedback our bodies constantly give us. No pain no gain. We go into nonstop war with the resistance we feel. So now we get to reconnect and relearn.

This means tuning in to how we feel, responding, and getting to know every inch of our bodies extremely well. We get to know ourselves by exploring: move easy, everything you've got, in every direction you can move it. Underlying this exploration are some key principles of movement that bring us back to nature—and along with it, back to being limitlessly capable in doing everything there is for us to do. No force, no struggle, no stress. Just feeling good the entire time. Which brings me to my principles of natural movement.

I gathered these principles from two decades of martial arts competition, where I got to see what worked and didn't work for a whole lot of people. Now I see people at yoga every day, and the same principles apply.

It's worth remembering that these are not simply techniques to learn and check off a list. Natural movement and its principles grow from an understanding of yourself—a way of being—that you can continue to discover and improve throughout your entire life.

Also, this is an all-day, everyday practice; it's not just for yoga class. Keep an eye on yourself in everything you do. See where you are working hard or not feeling good. Notice where you might be using force against resistance in your body or holding on to stress rather than letting it go. Then change it. Find a natural way to move where you aren't working so hard, a way that allows stress to leave your body and mind. Keep playing with this every chance you get.

We all have this wonderful human body. There isn't a single person I have ever met who is too big or too small, too short or too tall, too slow or too fast, overly bendy or underly flexible. Everybody has an advantage, to do whatever they need to do. You just need to find yours. You do this by finding yourself and connecting back to your nature.

So here they are: 11 principles to natural movement that will get you moving easily and powerfully, without tiring, in everything you do. You'll recognize some of these from the previous chapters, but since each chapter builds on the next, these are essential pieces of natural movement.

PRINCIPLE 1 Soften

If you are a solid-stone statue, all flexed, engaged, and ready to go, nothing that follows will work for you. Stone is immovable. Flexed and engaged muscles are immovable. It's never a good idea to immobilize yourself and then try to move. That's just frustrating. So as a start, see if you are soft enough to be movable.

Here's your softness test. When you move your middle, does the rest of your body—your arms and legs—go easily along for the ride? Or are you working hard to be where you are, so moving your middle has no effect on the rest of you?

If it's the first, you're ready to move. If it's the second, take a few deep breaths, put a little easy bend in your joints, and give your hips another wiggle to see where you are now.

Always make sure your body is soft and happily movable before you try to move. Moving becomes really easy and really fun this way.

PRINCIPLE 2 Establish Your Breath-Body Connection

Establishing your breath-body connection means that when you breathe, your body moves. Your inhales will begin an easy lifting and strengthening of your body; your exhales will soften and make you more movable.

The single hardest point of movement, from an energy perspective, is when you must overcome inertia to go from zero movement to movement. You can use your muscles to initiate this movement, but muscles get tired pretty quickly, so it's better to use your breath—it's the one thing you can do all day long without getting tired.

Have a seat, and get comfortable. Now take a really long, deep breath. If you're working hard to hold yourself where you are, not much will happen. If you're comfortable and relaxed, your breath will move you. You'll sit a little taller on your breath in, and a little softer on your breath out.

You can apply this to everything you do. From a comfortable and relaxed position, use every inhale to lift and strengthen your body and every exhale to release tension and make yourself movable.

PRINCIPLE 3 Lead from Your Middle

You can get your arms and legs to move by simply moving your arms and legs, or you can get them to move by moving first from your middle and letting the rest of you go along for the ride. The first way you'll work much harder than you need to and you'll tire out quickly. If you move from your middle, you'll be much more efficient, and you'll move faster and more powerfully without tiring.

Here's an experiment: Try standing with your feet two feet apart. Keep your legs flexed and your knees locked. Now swing your arms around just by moving your shoulders, while keeping your hips pointing straight forward.

Not fun at all, right?

Let it go! Take a deep breath. Relax your legs, put a little bend in your knees, and just let your arms hang easy. Now roll your belly and hips to point left, and right, and back left. Keep rolling side to side, letting your legs and arms just move how they want. You've movable, right from your middle, and the rest of your body just gets to go along for the ride.

Leading from your breath and your hips gives you a tireless source of movement, and it's much stronger and more effective than leading movement from your hands and feet.

PRINCIPLE 4 Use Your Opposites

Move away from your goal, then toward it.

If you want to go forward, first go back. Similarly, go back to go forward, up to go down, down to go up, left to go right, and right to go left.

Let's try it in a plank. Get into the top of your push-up position, with both your hands and feet about shoulder-width apart. Take a deep breath to lift your hips and body a little higher. Exhale and put a little bend in your elbows and knees.

To move from a plank to a side plank on your right hand, first go left. Gently lean your hips to the left as you inhale. Then exhale back through center, and let your hips go right as you inhale and roll onto your right hand into a side plank.

Try it a few times, and give yourself lots freedom to make bigger and bigger rocking movements. Want to get on your left hand? Rock to the right, then roll left into your side plank.

If you'd like to compare this with stressed, unnatural movement, here's a second experiment. Try moving from plank to side plank with all your joints locked tight and body stiff as a board, no rocking whatsoever. You'll likely discover it's more fun to rock.

PRINCIPLE 5 Use Momentum

Make friends with momentum. If you fight movement, you'll lose.

If you want to make some large, more challenging moves, first make some smaller moves to get your momentum going. Once your body is moving freely from side to side, forward and back, up and down, it's much easier to go where you want to go. By contrast, if you unnaturally immobilize, flex, and tense your body before attempting something challenging (like a handstand), it will just cause stress, and your movement will be much harder than it needs to be.

Try this in a single leg forward bend, moving toward a warrior 3. Start with one foot about four feet behind the other. Relax your legs, and put a good bend in both knees so your fingertips are comfortably on the ground, arms dropping straight down from your shoulders. Give your hips a wiggle and rock a little side to side, just to see that you're movable and relaxed. You always want to move from movable and relaxed! Now lean back into your back foot; then rock forward onto your front foot. Suddenly you're in warrior 3 without even trying.

Do this a few times, with a good bend in your knees, walking your hands back and then forward to support this movement. Now add your breath to the mix, inhaling as you lean back, exhaling as you rock through center, and inhaling to pull you all the way forward onto your front foot. It's all just one easy, continuous movement with your breath.

You can apply this same technique for rocking into a handstand. With your fingertips on the ground, come to a single leg forward bend with your back knee on the ground. Just sit comfortably on your back heel, keep your chest upright for this one, and take a few breaths. Now look forward and rock your whole body forward at once—hips, shoulders, hands all come forward. Your hands plant a couple of feet in front of your front foot, and your shoulders and hips will continue forward as you rock and lift gently toward a handstand. Now as you exhale, lower and rock yourself back to your starting point, relax, and repeat. Inhale rocks you forward; exhale relaxes you back.

PRINCIPLE 6 Use Your Whole Body

When meeting a challenge, get your whole body involved. Never isolate or immobilize one part while attempting to move another. Isolation leads to greatly reduced ability and eventually to injury. Whole-body unity leads to easy demolition of challenges.

Let's take push-ups as an example. Imagine (but avoid) holding a plank stiff and tense, arms and legs locked. Then lower halfway down, elbows by your sides directly over your wrists, shoulder blades engaged and drawing together. Now push straight back up and repeat, again, and again, and again. Remember, please don't do this! Even under the best conditions, it causes stress, reduced ability, and with enough repetition, repeat-use injury. Now let's look at why and how to make it better.

Generally immobilizing your body in a stiff plank pose, then lowering and lifting through push-ups by moving only your arms is just about the least capable and least valuable way you can do push-ups. You'll feel a great deal of effort and fatigue in your shoulders and arms, because they are doing nearly all the work. In the rest of your body, if you feel anything, it will just be stress from holding tension while you do your push-ups. This is the best way to tire yourself out quickly and accomplish less with more effort. Now let's try something different.

Start in a plank pose. First, let's get movable. Widen your hands and feet to mat width, and soften your elbows and knees, allowing the joints to bend easily. Now that you have a stable and movable base, let's move. Rock your hips gently side to side, and then make those rocks big enough that your hands and feet move around a bit—not because you're trying to move them, but because you're moving your body from your middle, and they are eventually attached to your middle. So now you know your body is ready to move. So let's move.

Take a big inhale to lift your hips a bit, then long exhale as you ease your whole body toward the floor; roll around from side to side as you come down to your belly. Now keep rolling around from side to side as an inhale lifts your hips and body back up to the ceiling, and repeat.

You might be leaning more on one hand or the other, one foot or the other might be on or off the ground, or off to the side, or a little closer to your hands. Your whole body is movable and moving freely along for this ride as you lift and lower. Is it challenging? Of course! But it's your whole body in on it, continuously adapting to move in its own most capable way. Stress never has a chance to build in any one part of you, and you'll be able to do far more with far less effort.

The same works for handstands. Often I see people planting their palms, locking their arms, shoulders, and upper bodies as if fixed in concrete, then swinging one leg repeatedly to the sky, with the hope of launching into a handstand. This leg-swinging exercise might occasionally lead to a handstand, or to crashing over backward, or simply to falling right back down. In each of these scenarios, the strength of one kicking leg must be absorbed by resistance in your shoulders and wrists. Eventually, the wrists and shoulders lose in this conflict. Handstands might happen here, but with the most possible effort, and without the coordination and grace that can lead to so much more than just a handstand. So let's find a better way.

Come into a comfortable runner's stretch, right foot forward, with your left knee on the ground, back toes tucked, and sitting easily on your back heel. Keep your body relaxed, up and open, rather than in a forward fold, and your fingertips resting on the ground. Get comfortable here, rocking gently hand to hand, just to make sure your body is relaxed enough to be movable. Now let's move!

Walk your hands forward, letting your hips and whole body follow, until your hands are two or three feet in front of your front foot. Plant your palms here, and let your shoulders and hips keep rolling forward over your hands until there is no more weight on your left foot. Your right knee is bent and your hips are rolling open as the weight gently comes out of your left foot, so you just bend your left knee to lift the foot from the ground. Then as you exhale, let your left foot down and roll easily back to your runner's stretch, and repeat. Let this be a continuous motion with your breath. Your whole body rolling forward, planting your palms, and still rolling forward and open over your hands until there is no weight on your standing leg. Then your whole body relaxing all the way back. There is no kicking leg involved here, no use of force against some resistant or tense part of your body. You won't even realize you are working hard, because everything in you is working easily together, as a single whole. You have achieved oneness!

Always handle everything you can in this way. Use your whole body to open doors, lift objects, and move every part of you in your yoga practice. Anytime you notice some part of you not moving while other parts are moving, free that immovable part. Drop the tension, and get your whole body moving naturally together again. You'll accomplish far more in this way, without even realizing that what you are doing is hard.

PRINCIPLE 7 Open the Door, Close the Door

When you approach a challenge, always move from where you are comfortable, open, and feeling good. If you are already uncomfortable before you move further into a challenge, it won't get any better. From uncomfortable, your ability to move happily and easily will progressively decline, and you will be left with only a single option: using pure force to overcome resistance.

Imagine the following scenario, preferably without actually doing it, because it's an example of what not to do! Sink into a deep chair pose, and hold here for several breaths. From this deep chair, pick up your right foot and cross your right ankle over your left knee, so you're now in a hip opener, with your left knee still deeply bent. Keeping your left knee deeply bent, now hook your right elbow on the bottom of your right foot. Hold for a few breaths. Now bend your left knee even deeper, twist your body toward the left, and place both palms on the ground, shoulder-width apart, to the left of your left foot. Tip over into an arm balance, with your right knee and foot pressing into your right upper arm. Hold for a bit; then shoot back into a push-up. Remember, this an example of what not to do. Now let's examine why, and how to make it better.

For a long time, it was believed in yoga that burning through this kind of progressive discomfort was a valuable path to purification and transcendence. But the science of stress has come a long way, and it's now clear that this just isn't a good idea. There are many benefits to developing focus, and simply moving our bodies, that might make any yoga better than doing nothing. But furthering our chemical addiction to our body's stress response, by putting even more stress in our yoga, isn't the best we can do. We can do much better.

This is where "Open the Door, Close the Door" comes in. Always open the door to movement first so you don't have to force your way through. Create room and comfort in your body, and then move into a challenge from a space of comfort. Then reopen the door and move again into challenge. When your body is challenged or compressed—for example, with strong muscular effort or difficult twists—the door begins to close: moving deeper into a pose from here will cause stress and declining ability. So rather than run into a closed door again and again, as with the example above, we always reopen the door, releasing stress before moving into additional challenge.

Let's try this, taking chair pose and twisting chair pose as an example. From a standing forward fold, start to sink your hips as you roll up to a chair. Let a big inhale lift you up out of this chair, a long exhale as you lower and twist to the right, another big inhale pulls you up to a lifted chair, a long exhale to lower and twist to the left, a big inhale to lift back through center, and a big exhale to dive over and hang easy in a forward fold. With each movement here, you use your inhale to open the door, creating space and comfort in your body, and you exhale to move into compression or challenge, then another inhale to lift you back to open.

High lunge twists work similarly. Start in a high lunge with your right foot forward. Take a long inhale to lift your high lunge—as long as you're breathing in, you're lifting your hips and floating straight up. There is space and comfort in your body here. The door is open. Then as you exhale, roll your belly toward the right and soften into a nice twist. Your hips are sinking as you roll to the right, into a compressed and more challenged position. Then let your next inhale pull you back up into a lifted high lunge.

From here you have a choice. The door is open. So your next exhale could bring you to another twist, or it could bring you to another open position, rolling your back heel down, and softening into a warrior 2. The only thing that doesn't happen is that when the door is closed—in a compressed or challenged position—you don't move into a more compressed or more challenged position. It's unnatural to move into a closed door. It leads to more stress, declining ability to move, and increased likelihood of injury. So keep opening doors. Always move into challenges from where you are comfortable and open.

PRINCIPLE 8 Conserve Energy

Use just enough effort to do what is needed—nothing more, nothing less.

I see so many people holding simple poses, like warrior 2, flexing every muscle as hard as they can. The idea is that if you work very hard here, you might build more strength to eventually handle greater challenges. It's a nice theory, but I've never seen it work—for anyone. If you practice working harder than you need to while doing simple things, you will simply get good at working harder than you need to. This creates a glass ceiling for your abilities, in yoga and everything else. When more complex challenges come up, you will be good at working harder than you need, which makes it impossible to do anything that is actually hard or complex.

Exhausting ourselves while doing even simple things might also seem appealing because it can have a nice, sedating effect on our minds. But there are better ways for this. There's really never a need to think about exercising yourself. You'll get very strong, and very movable, just by moving in natural response to what's in front of you. Not too much, not too little, just right.

You'll find that your body is extremely well designed to do what is needed, in any situation—from the most simple to the most challenging. Similarly, you'll find that your body is very poorly designed to work harder than is needed. The result is declining ability and eventually injury and poor health.

This is an important one in nature. A tree never works harder than needed to stand or reach the light. It simply does what it needs to do. The wind blows, and it sways, just enough. The light is blocked, so it grows toward the light, just enough. In the same way, you won't find a tiger exercising itself. It will not tire out its mind thinking about flexing, engaging, extending, or rotating when it climbs a tree. The tiger simply climbs the tree. It simply moves, using just enough effort to do what is needed, no more and no less. Nature always conserves energy in this way, existing in just the right balance between strength and flexibility, stability, and mobility.

The same is true when humans are working optimally. Did you ever see Michael Jordan play basketball? When he decided to drive the hoop, he just went. Feet on or off the ground, it didn't much matter. Now imagine if he had to stop first, flex his arms, engage his thighs, pull in his belly, and rotate his shoulders. Not much would happen from here! The same goes for any top-performing athlete. Natural movement always beats unnatural movement. When we're working optimally, we don't work harder than we need. In fact, we don't even think about how much we're working. We just move. We do exactly what it takes to get it done.

Does this mean we never fire it up and get that great burn? Not exactly. If you're training to win an Olympic sprint, play professional rugby, or fight with bears, then yes, you need to build a great deal of raw power, agility, and endurance to handle far greater challenges than are in most everyday routines. But even here, as the challenges grow, you never work harder than needed. You keep growing with the challenges you face, and doing exactly what is needed to handle them. In this way, we can all become extremely capable in our own bodies, at every level of performance.

PRINCIPLE 9 Sensitize

Move how it feels good to move. Adjust the path you take from one point to another—including direction, angle of approach, speed, acceleration, and deceleration—based on the signals your body sends to you in each moment.

Tune every inch of your movement to what's going on in your body and how every part of you is relating to every other part, in this moment. How? It's those three steps we discussed in Chapter 3: slow down, believe, respond. Let's do a quick recap here.

STEP 1: SLOW DOWN. At least some of the time, move slowly enough and breathe deeply enough that you have a chance to feel every inch that you move through. Your body is always sending you signals about how things are working. Give yourself a chance to notice them.

STEP 2: BELIEVE. You need to believe that how you feel is worth responding to. This is a big one. We're so often used to ignoring how we feel and pushing through discomfort that we pay no attention to what our bodies are saying. This approach might work occasionally and temporarily, but it's not the best way.

Ignoring and pushing through discomfort is a form of suboptimal movement. You're overriding your body's signals to achieve temporary gain. Your body will put up with this, but only for a while. You are only designed to move this way in case of extreme need or danger. Continued operation in this manner leads to declining mobility, reduced agility and endurance, and a higher likelihood of injury. So there must be a better way, one that fits with your natural design.

Here's the better way: believe that when something doesn't feel good, you should find a different way to move. This will make the next step possible.

STEP 3: RESPOND. You're feeling and believing that what you feel is relevant to your progress. Now respond. You'll feel a bit different from one side of your body to the other, and from one day to the next. So how you move each day, how you move on each side, will be a bit different, if you're responding to the signals your body is sending.

If something hurts or feels stuck—resistant to movement—this is a signal that there's a better way. Find the ways to do what you need to do that feel best. When something doesn't feel good, steer around it. Choose a slightly different route, approach angle, speed, acceleration, or deceleration to get where you want to go. When something feels good, almost effortless compared with the other way, you've found it.

PRINCIPLE 10 Focus on Body Position

If softness is the beginning, the soul, of natural movement, body position is its heart. With optimal body position—all your parts in just the right position relative to all your other parts—you can move easily, quickly, and powerfully, with little effort. Without it, many things will be harder, and some will be impossible, even unimaginable. It's how the old tai chi master gently reminds the young Olympic competitor that there is something more than the accumulation of techniques here.

Discovering and using your best body position carries across everything you do. Your stance—where you place your hands, feet, arms, legs, everything—is the base for how you will move, how much effort it will require, and how much you'll be able to accomplish from where you are.

Imagine putting yourself in a high lunge. In your mind, make it extralong front to back, and bend your front knee deep, so it is aligned directly above your ankle, and the top of your thigh is parallel to the ground. Now go to a warrior 3.

That's hard to do, isn't it? It would take a great deal of strain, and likely you would need to kick off with your back foot to propel yourself forward.

So it's possible to do this. But it's not a good idea. In this imaginary setting, you've used force to overcome resistance in your body—the strength of kicking your back thigh against reluctance in your knee. That kick forces your deeply bent front knee forward of your ankle, subjecting it to even more stress than it already had in its nicely aligned but still-strained position. You'll work much harder than you need to, which leads to injury and the ability to do much less than your true capacity allows.

Now imagine something different. You're in a high lunge, but it's shorter from front to back, and your back knee is softly bent. Now inhale to lift your hips and body high, exhale to lean a little weight into your back foot, and inhale to roll your belly forward. The rest of your body—chest, arms, legs—will go along for the ride. Your front knee will have never moved while deeply bent and challenged. It will also have remained safely above the ankle throughout the whole movement. You'll be in warrior 3 thinking you've done not much more than breathe your way into it. Which is true.

But is this possible? Have we cheated in some way? This has been hard for years, and suddenly now it just isn't hard anymore, so how could that be right? Yet we've done the same movement, accomplished the same work, and have energy in our bodies for far more than we ever imagined possible.

This is the power of natural movement. This is your power.

PRINCIPLE 11 Play

Have fun with what you're doing. Remember, you're here to feel and find your way to feeling good.

Adults are too good at immobilizing themselves and then trying to move. We're too good at making easy things hard, and we put too low a ceiling on our own potential in this way.

To unlearn this, remember what it was like to play. Then play. No thinking. Let your mind go. Have fun with you.

When you're playing Frisbee, or driving for the hoop, you don't need to think about any of these natural movement principles. When you're having fun, when you're playing happily in your body, your nature takes over. You don't have to think about your yoga or your sport; you just feel it. You just do it.

The principles of natural movement can help when we find ourselves in the middle of something new, unfamiliar, or less comfortable. But even here, put joy in it. Put joy in every single thing you do. Even the hard things. Keep them playful. Keep joy in being you, every move, everywhere. It's the number one principle to move inspiringly as an athlete. And it's the number one principle to move inspiringly in your life.

ROUNDING OUT NATURAL MOVEMENT

As you've seen, you can do easy things the hard way, or hard things the easy way. Moving with tension in our bodies and minds is unnatural for us—it causes stress and makes everything much harder than it needs to be. We might achieve some challenges by forcing things this way, but we probably won't enjoy it that much. It just doesn't feel good.

It's better to do hard things the easy way. From here we can do far more, with far less effort. And fortunately, it's in our nature.

The world is full of tension and stress, unnatural rules, and constraints. But we can learn to change it. We can remember that we are not stuck.

We make this change first inside. Not by saying, "The world is just hard and doesn't feel good, so we need to endure it." But by saying that we create this world—and we can re-create it, first in our own bodies and minds and then the rest of it. We can practice this in our yoga. We can put it in our lives.

So if we're going to get good at something, maybe it shouldn't be the common yoga practice of enduring strain and stress. Maybe the one thing you should get good at is you. Not someone else's techniques, someone else's rules, shapes, or ideas. Your shape, your way. You. This doesn't come from someone else, a teacher, a guru. It comes from you connecting to you—your nature—learning to feel and respond to what you feel.

By putting natural movement in your life, you are never out of alignment with yourself. You don't make problems to fix. You are in this way always in the right place for you. From here, you get very good at working with everything you've got, which makes it a whole lot easier to do everything there is.

When you get good at you, you get good at everything. You create you exactly how you want, from here. You create the world how you want from here.

Now that you've gotten to know a bit more about the Strala philosophy—and you've experienced it in your own life—let's move on to Part II of the book: how to orchestrate this experience for other people.

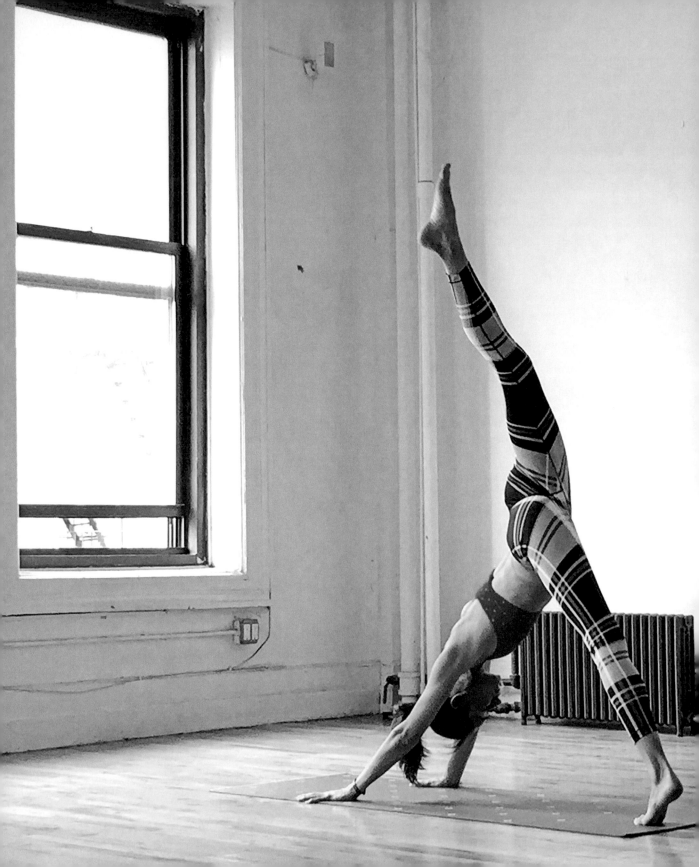

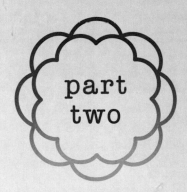

part
two

orchestrate

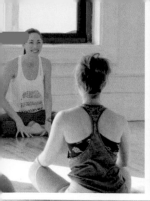

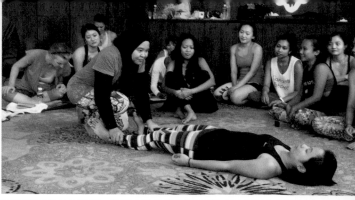
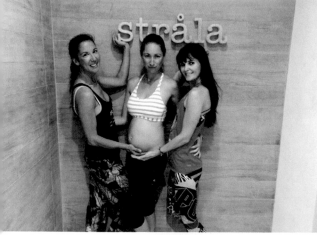
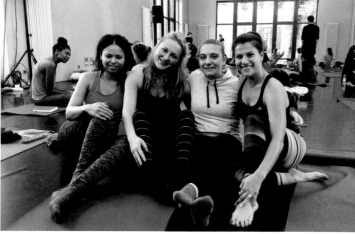
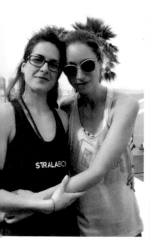

> **"**
> Asking someone how they feel may just lighten their load by a whole lot.
> **"**

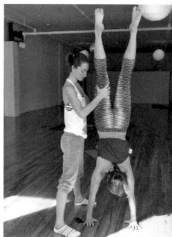
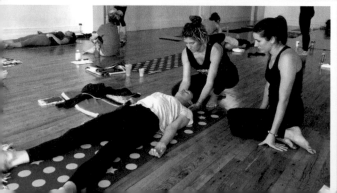
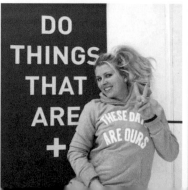

THE STRALA OUTLOOK

CREATING A SUPPORTIVE ENVIRONMENT

Bringing Strala to others is all about creating an internal experience for them. Everything we do is an effort to bring people more deeply into their minds and their bodies so they can access the innate knowledge that will help them thrive in life. So many yoga classes are focused on the external—mastering poses, getting a workout, trying to look your best. But Strala is all about going inside.

The process of guiding an internal experience comes from everywhere: your guiding, your voice, your language, your tone, your ability to touch people in a nonthreatening way—all those things that most people don't think about when they think about a class. These intangibles are sensed. They are the things that make people feel good—or not so good in some instances.

In any given class, Strala draws a wide range of people with different backgrounds, ages, experiences, and bodies—and that's because we're known for our focus on the internal. We don't push. We don't judge. We don't do anything other than encourage people to be who they are, right here, right now. The focus is them. This begins when your guest walks through the front door, is welcomed by you, and enters the space. And it continues with everything that goes into your leading of the class. Everything you do should be done in an effort to make people feel welcomed and empowered to move, feel, and heal.

WHY EASE?

The main ingredient in helping people tap into themselves is exploring in an environment of ease. Our goal as Guides is to create a feeling of ease in every interaction we have. This requires a lot of focus, attention, and care, so it's important that you truly understand why it matters. If you understand, on a gut level, why an easy and open experience is necessary, your efforts to create it won't be as difficult, which means you're more likely to do it.

So I'd like you to take some time right now and really think about it. What are the benefits of an easeful atmosphere? When you've considered it for a bit, grab your journal and write down anything that came to mind, even if it seems silly. And then let's compare notes!

Here are some of the reasons that I think creating ease all around is important:

1. An environment of ease helps people breathe deeper and more freely.

2. An easygoing atmosphere creates less tension in the body and creates a safe environment that promotes healing.

3. People feel welcome and relaxed.

4. People feel like they can be themselves.

5. People feel free to ask questions before and after class.

6. As the Guide an environment of ease helps people understand that I am there to help them.

7. An easygoing environment is open and clear of clutter, which promotes an internal experience.

8. People are able to accomplish more with less effort because of the lack of tension.

You'll discover loads about yourself by examining your thoughts and actions as you create your guiding experience. You'll get more information and inspiration about how you'd like to help people and all the ways you can create the optimal environment to serve. Every little thing matters, and the more we pay attention to the details of how we are and what we are doing, the better we can help ourselves and others.

EASE BEGINS WITH YOU

You may have noticed that I said that you should aim to create ease in every interaction. I wasn't kidding. This needs to happen for the people not only in your classes and one-on-one sessions but also, more broadly, in any moment in life. I can't say this enough: you give others the experience of who you are. Understanding how you affect others will shift you. It will help you lean in to guiding people to connect to themselves whether you are leading a yoga class, having a conversation, or taking a deep breath around a tense situation. Guiding ease in a yoga class is only possible when you constantly participate in the process of ease regularly for yourself.

Strala, along with many other things in life, works only when you experience, understand, and decide for yourself that the approach works. Simply memorizing language, concepts, and movement phrases will not lead to a great-feeling class. Understanding *how* and *why* these elements work and why they lead to a great feeling will make your classes feel uniquely special. Owning the leading for yourself will create the experience that feels like you.

When you guide from a clear understanding, you will shine through the experience. People will be drawn to the unique qualities you possess that make you a fantastic Guide and healer. The Guide is the most important element to the class. You are what the experience ultimately feels like. When you simply memorize what to do and regurgitate the system robotically, people will never be able to experience your greatness and the experience will always fall flat.

ENCOURAGING PRACTICE

While you are the most important element of creating an easeful environment, you must remember that you are not the most important person in the class. The goal of creating ease is to create a space where others feel comfortable and empowered to find themselves.

Part of our job as Guides is to encourage people to practice. Obviously we do this by being a wonderful example of radiant well-being and ease, but this doesn't always cut it for those people who have misconceptions about what yoga is or should be. Which means that you need to be equipped to handle the resistance that comes your way with joy and ease.

Here are some common misconceptions, excuses, and practical reasons why many people don't practice:

❋ I'm not flexible.

❋ I have to be more in shape before I start yoga.

❋ I got injured from a yoga class and I'm not going back.

❋ Yoga is boring.

❋ Yoga is too hard.

❋ It's too hot in that room.

❋ I don't want to chant something I don't understand.

❋ I don't want to spend my hour I have for myself getting lectured.

I've heard all of these comments—and so many more—so many times. While there are millions of people practicing yoga now, the majority of people are not, so there is still a lot of work for us to do. And we're not just trying to convince the unconvinced to start a yoga practice; we're also trying to inspire people from other, more externally focused practices to look within.

To do this, it's nice to have easy answers for every excuse you may get—and these answers can be found in an easygoing approach that focuses on the person where they are right now.

Can't touch your toes? No problem. Just bend your knees. The goal isn't to be a contortionist; it's about creating healthy mobility for longevity, so we can feel better. Yoga is boring? Maybe you had a funny experience. What happened? Yoga is too hard? Show with your class that it is possible to face challenges in an easygoing way that will ignite the relaxation response so you feel great during the whole process. Don't want a lecture? No problem. We stay with the practice and leave room for you to be you. The easygoing approach won't give you the workout you want? Just try it.

More impactful than going on the defense against the yoga resistant is coming back to that circle of being. What you choose to convey—through your actions and your words—about the benefits they will experience helps convince people more than anything else. Contradict their excuse while reminding them that they will feel better, pain-free, sensitized to their bodies and minds, calm, and expansive. Remind them that they're not there to do poses. They're there to feel. Everything good they can imagine comes from this.

MAKE IT ABOUT THEM

Once people have experienced the process, our goal is to keep them engaged. One of the ways to do this is to keep the classes interesting, and the way to do this is to be interested in people. As Guides, we aim to connect and support, not change, control, and manipulate. If you can become fascinated with all different kinds of people and build a healthy relationship with your ability to relate to others, people will be happy to be around you. I emphasize becoming fascinated with different kinds of people because who you care about is who gravitates toward you. To keep a diverse and interesting class of people, you have to care about diverse and interesting people. You need to make everyone feel welcome.

I have a simple policy to do this. I use it myself and with the Strala Guides I train around the world. Make yourself available and focus your attention on anyone who comes in.

When someone walks into the studio, simply say hi and ask how they're doing. The simplicity of the greeting directs the attention to the guest and puts the Guide in the supporting role. This focus allows us to gather the information about our guests that will facilitate a great experience. By being welcoming and hospitable, we open the floor for our guests to share how they are doing, if anything is bothering them, if anything is especially great, or if something out of the ordinary is happening. This process creates ease and space for our guests to feel welcome and safe.

I'll take this one step further and share a little trick that helps people relax, open up, and start the process of ease. If a guest asks me how I am doing or what I've been up to lately, I'll answer politely, but soon I'll turn the attention back on them. Something like, "Oh, I just got back from London. It was fun to do classes with everyone there. What have you been up to?" I avoid going on and on about myself, my day, and my ideas, and by doing so I create space for my guest. It's part of the magic of creating an internal experience of ease for yourself and for those around you.

If I haven't had a chance to greet everyone, I make sure to find an opportunity to do so in class, whether it's through eye contact or touch. I try to connect with everyone because I know that it feels nice to be acknowledged by the host of the experience.

A Guide can gain a following by going on and on about themselves in a charismatic way day after day, but that process misses the real potential of helping people get in touch with themselves. A self-indulgent attitude creates a following of people who ultimately idolize the leader. A welcoming attitude creates a following of people who return to the experience because they are inspired to connect with themselves. The welcoming approach is everlasting, powerful, transformational, and strong. The self-indulgent may accomplish temporary excitement, but ultimately, idols fall and people look for the next new thing. Do yourself a favor on your journey of guiding. Open the stage, turn the light toward your guests, and get interested in who they are. You'll help more efficiently and feel energized and rewarded.

EYES, EARS & BODY

Connecting with people is about so much more than asking them questions about themselves and their days. Even if you say, "How are you?" the experience depends on how this interaction occurs. If you stay seated on a bench, looking at your phone as you ask, it feels extremely different for the person you're talking to. If you get up, put your phone down, and really tune in to what they're saying, people feel the love and get comfortable. It's all about connection, the first piece of which comes from something as simple as eye contact.

The eyes are powerful tools. Giving someone your full attention by looking in their eyes when they speak feels different than if you're staring at the floor or looking at someone or something else in the room. Eye contact can create a feeling of camaraderie before, during, and after class. While looking everyone in the eyes when you lead might be overwhelming, it's important to do it sometimes—especially if you're trying to relay something to someone in particular. Use your sense of judgment and instinct with the intention of welcoming and helping, without invading people's personal space and calm.

In my personal experience, catching someone's eye while leading class can be wonderful and supportive, but it's nice when it happens naturally and isn't sought out for the whole class. I like to think of eye contact when leading as hot sauce. It's a wonderful and powerful ingredient when you use it appropriately and sparingly.

Listening intently is the next piece of creating a connection. What you don't say can be even more important than what you do say. It's amazing how healing it can be for someone to have you listen to her, instead of interrupting quickly with advice. Think of a time when you really wanted to talk to a good friend about a problem. Did your friend solve your problem for you? Did he go out and fix the situation and make everything magically better?

If your friend was able to help you feel better, he probably accomplished that by simply listening. We solve our own problems, come to our own solutions in what action we need to take. We don't do this alone, however. In human connection, we allow space for healing. When a friend hugs us when we are down, we feel better. It's not because she has magical healing powers in her hands and arms. It's because she is bringing her whole self to us and offering support. This is where it gets really cool. Your friends are actually leaning on and being supported by you! Healing takes place when we are able to give and receive with our whole selves. Providing a healing environment happens when we are able to bring our whole selves to the other person, and often lean on him physically and emotionally for support.

How you hold yourself is another incredibly powerful tool that might not be so obvious unless you spend time in practice and self-care. If you are hunched forward with your arms crossed as you listen to or speak with someone, or if you're fidgeting with your hands and feet, your energy is muddled and you appear distracted, or not interested. The same goes when leading class. We practice with the same point of view when it comes to leading. Soften the whole body and the whole self as you move around and navigate the room. Present yourself as open. Arms relaxed and easy, posture tall and calm, breath full and deep, eyes clear and curious, ready to help. With regular practice and attention, you can always improve your body language. If you don't pay any attention to it, it will continue to be as it is, which might not be so bad, but to ignore a powerful tool when it comes to presenting your whole self would be a big miss.

EXPLAINING STRALA—OR NOT

Another element of keeping people engaged is to focus on the experience itself. The magic of your class lies in the experience. It's not necessary to explain all the ingredients and purposes intellectually to people before they practice.

In fact, doing so would take away from the openness and uniqueness of the experience. So in Strala, we don't explain when we guide; we lead and allow the experience to speak for itself.

I like to explain the importance of firsthand experience in terms of food—because who doesn't love food? Imagine trying your favorite dish for the first time. You don't know it's your favorite until you try. The chef presents the dish to you, knowing the goodness that went into creating it. He smiles with care, places the plate in front of you, and lets you enjoy that first bite. He doesn't tell you about all the ingredients. He doesn't explain why the sweet and the tart work together. He doesn't tell you about how the smell affects your salivary glands. He knows all this, but he simply lets you taste the food and experience the joy it provides.

Think of yourself as the chef of the Strala experience. Let the person take that first bite and enjoy. If she wants to, she can come to you to share, ask questions, and get all the secret ingredients. There is no need to explain the yoga before leading the yoga. Getting out of the intellect and into the experience is a big part of creating space for healing—and the feelings of well-being and health will keep people coming back.

Focusing on doing also creates a community that inspires ease and practice. Many people quite naturally come together after class to discuss what they experienced. Doing this in a casual setting can be useful, especially when someone is dealing with a specific ailment, injury, or emotional situation. So leave space for people to interact before and after class, but never force a lecture or take the stage to explain. It's powerful to allow space for people to experience the class and let them feel and process however they like. The choice is theirs to give you feedback, share how great they feel, or talk about the philosophy in more detail. We are simply, and profoundly, Guides.

GUIDE VERSUS TEACHER

Keeping people engaged is encouraged by anything we do to help them tap into their own power. You may or may not have noticed that I've been using the term *Guide* instead of *teacher* throughout this book. This is intentional. Language is a powerful influencer in people's experiences, and focusing on guiding rather than teaching is a crucial part of this.

When I started guiding yoga, I was extremely passionate about people's power to connect to their bodies' innate knowledge in order to heal. I knew that this process was best guided, not instructed. The hierarchy presented by the teacher-student relationship also seemed incredibly silly to me. I was a young adult with a passion for and knowledge of yoga. I was eager to help others connect, but I was no expert on the people around me. They simply needed to plug back into themselves. I couldn't teach them, but I could share my experiences. I could share what I'd seen in others. I was there simply as a source of information that they could use as they searched out their own unique path to peace and health.

I also had a fundamental problem with the connotations brought on by the word *teacher*. For someone to be a teacher, it implies that he has something that you don't and you have to go through him to get it. He is the expert; you are not. He can tell you when you are right or wrong; you have no say in it. When we are in primary school simply collecting facts and learning about the world around us, the word *teacher* is acceptable. Reading, writing, and math are pretty cut-and-dried. But when we engage in learning about our emotions and our mind-body connection, there is nobody better than you to lead your exploration. You are the world's leading expert on you. When you let someone else lead your exploration, you give away your power and often you don't move forward as quickly or as beneficially.

The other thing I didn't like about using the word *teacher* was that it implies a strict relationship of passing along facts. There is no expectation that a teacher will share a part of herself with the people in class. The uninterested math teacher staring at the blackboard while writing out problems and solutions seems to be something many of us can call to mind. Of course, our most memorable teachers are the ones that go above and beyond simply presenting information. They embody attention, live in the present, believe in us, and inspire us to believe in ourselves. These teachers have moved into what I believe is the realm of Guide.

In Strala Yoga, we use the term *Guide* to return power to the people in our classes. We do not put ourselves above anyone else. We do not hold ourselves up as authorities. As Guides we have knowledge when it comes to a process, we have experience in the practice, and we have a sense that everyone is on their own journey. They are doing the work; we are simply there to lend a hand. Just as a guide would do in mountain climbing. A careful climber enlists the help of a guide to improve safety and to get advice and knowledge from someone who has done a particular climb many times before—and has hopefully guided others safely on the journey.

GUIDE (N):
A person who advises or shows the way to others.

TEACHER (N):
A person who teaches or instructs, especially as a profession.

A Strala Guide has know-how, skill, and experience to keep people safe and lead them through an appropriate journey with the goal of connecting to themselves.

Giving up that potential authority is helpful to students and also hugely liberating for you. If you put yourself in a position of power, you may become addicted to the feelings associated with it, and you may fear that the old story of the student surpassing the teacher will come to pass. If you are living in this world of competition, you limit your ability to help people and you constantly worry, which leads to stress and frustration. Hold power over others, and you'll never be full. You'll always be vulnerable to tension, self-judgment, and emotional imprisonment. Return the power to everyone, and become fully empowered.

The other term we use when referring to class is *leading*. We lead; we don't teach. The challenge this holds is that of embodying the philosophy yourself. You lead the process and the mind-set by being an example to everyone in your classes.

TEACH (V):
To impart knowledge or skill in, give instruction in.

LEAD (V):
To conduct by guiding, or show the way.

The goal of this philosophy and this language is to evolve past a dogmatic approach and empower people to sensitize themselves *to* themselves so they can live their fullest lives. Our goal is to help them look within—not out—for the answers. It's what all the yoga texts say, but somehow we lost the honor of the message in the evolution of its practice, an almost inevitable bump in the timeline of a system containing so much raw power. We're not here to criticize the service of teachers and those who teach; we're here to reshape the way we help others through the art of yoga and healing. It's essential to return the power to the practitioner, with experienced guidance, and dissolve invoking rituals by self-appointed gurus once and for all.

CREATING AN ENVIRONMENT OF EASE

I recently had someone apply to work at the Strala studio in New York City. As part of the interview, I asked a simple question that I like to ask anyone affiliated with Strala as a Guide or administrator: Why do you want to be here? The candidate told me she really liked how relaxed and open the environment felt and was looking for a job she could relax in—a job that would be easy. That told me she wasn't the right one for the position.

Creating an environment of ease doesn't mean we get to kick our feet up, space out, and chill. It means we spend a great deal of effort and attention creating and looking after ourselves and our environment so people can come in, feel welcomed, be themselves, and be at ease while working through simple and challenging moments. Being a provider of ease is a magical job. When you put careful attention on each moment, people feel at home in themselves, with you, and in the space. This means that they are simmering in an optimal space for lasting transformation.

It's important, this whole ease thing. I hope I got you on board to hold the space and deliver the magic. Remember, everything gets easier with practice, so try the following experiments in your daily life and see how your experience shifts.

1. When someone asks you how you are, answer honestly, and then ask him how he is. Follow up with more questions and take a genuine interest in what he says. Avoid pointing the conversation back to yourself. Keep the spotlight on your guest and stay interested.

2. Clean up clutter in your space, whether it's your home, workplace, or yoga studio. Set things up as if the most important person you can imagine is coming over. Treat yourself and your environment as if you were welcoming this person at any moment.

3. Offer your help to someone who needs it. Open a door when you're entering a store. Look around to see if anyone else is trying to get in. Treat the people you encounter as if they each were very important people you respect.

4. Smile more and mean it.

Everything you do to create ease in your own experiences will create ease for others. The more we practice, the more we improve, and we can all improve throughout our lives. Leading yoga holds the responsibility of being an example of a compassionate, thoughtful person, as well as leading a safe, productive, and expansive experience for a person or a group.

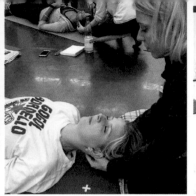
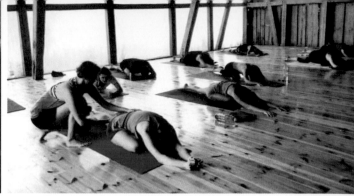
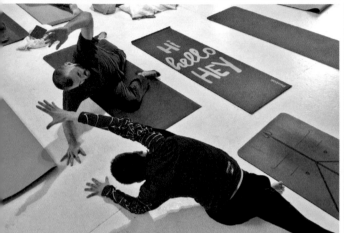

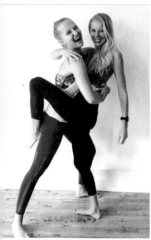
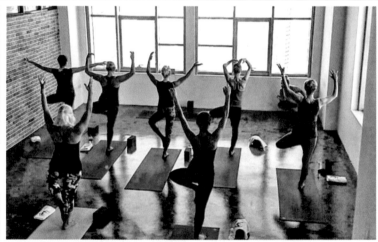
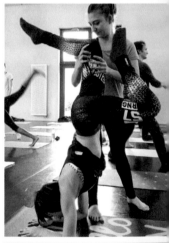
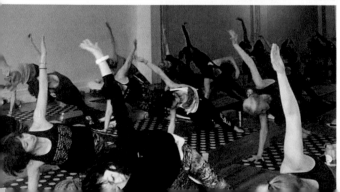
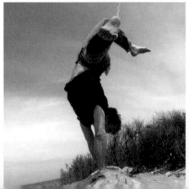

chapter
6

SETTING THE STAGE

CREATING A WELCOMING SPACE

Okay, so we've discussed the attitude and focus necessary to create an environment of ease, but what about the actual physical space—and all those "business" things associated with a studio? The experience people have in class begins long before they step on the mat for the first three breaths. From the moment a new person has heard about your class, she makes a judgment about you and your studio. How you greet people, how the space looks, the temperature, the cleanliness, the lighting, the smells, and the stuff in the room—everything matters.

GETTING THE WORD OUT

The process of telling people about your class can be one of the first impressions you make on them. How you communicate with people before you meet them in person matters. Did you get the word out about your class with flyers in the neighborhood or on social media? Or is greeting people in the space your first moment of impression? If you work for a gym, club, or studio, this may be the case. It's also possible that your first impression on people is simply word of mouth about the amazing work you're doing. If you do a good job at sharing positive concepts about your views on yoga and your classes, people might show up with the specific purpose of taking *your* class.

However you choose to do it, getting the word out is essential. If people can see the excitement you have for this process, they are more likely to come. If you do nothing to invite people to your classes, you're missing an opportunity—even if you believe it is someone else's responsibility to spread the word. You need to share information about your class in some way, whether through meeting people in person or digitally. In this day and age, there are so many choices for how to spend that hour or so a day on exercise and self-care. It's vital you do everything you can to get people to your classes—but it's critical not to alienate them while doing so.

As you're planning your outreach, try to be authentic and have a genuine positive attitude of wanting to help. Invite people with the attitude of taking care of them. Your class is an extension of that care. The last thing that people want is to feel bullied or guilt-tripped into coming. I've seen all kinds of approaches and a lot of variety in personalities over the years, and the Guides who build a positive, sustainable experience and the happiest regulars are the ones with the attitude of genuinely wanting to help people and an understanding that through helping, we feel a great sense of reward.

If that is missing from you, get out now. Find something else that makes your heart sing, and enjoy a different path. The world needs leaders of yoga who want to help.

CREATE SPACE . . . LITERALLY

So now on to the space itself. The space, whether it's your own studio, a gym, an event space, or a park, is a huge aspect of the class experience. How the space looks and feels matters a great deal. It could be the make-it-or-break-it piece that helps people feel at ease and dissolves stress, so they can naturally flow into the class comfortable, open, and with a calm and clear mind.

While we may not be able to find what we would consider the perfect room for practice, there is so much you can do with any space to create the best environment possible. It takes a great deal of attention to detail, creativity, and mindfulness to transform a space. Sometimes it's as simple as choosing which direction to face the class. Sometimes it's about removing clutter and cleaning. Whether you have control over the look and feel or are in a temporary space or working in another studio or gym, there are many things that factor into the experience your guests have.

In my New York studio, I'm adamant about the environment being clean, uncluttered, and open before anyone enters for class—these are things we can easily control. So each morning we clear any clutter, sweep the floor, arrange the fans, and ventilate the air as needed. We do this ourselves, every day. It's part of the normalcy that keeps things feeling nice. We don't hire cleaners or maids because we feel that it's important for us to be the ones cleaning and organizing. The space feels the best and most comfortable when you do the work yourself. It sets the stage for it to feel like a home. And we invite our guests into the space as if it were their home away from home. It's a special place set up to facilitate an experience of ease. Our guests can tangibly feel the good vibes and notice when we pick up the things to make it nice for them. This action creates the environment for good behavior from our guests, as well.

People regularly comment on how great the space feels. They often wonder if the feeling comes from the dimensions of the room, the number of windows, or the lighting. What makes it feel so good? I always let our guests believe whatever they want, because no matter what they think, they're right. Keeping the space cared for and filled with love opens people up to find the joy in whichever element speaks to them. The space feels great because of the careful, loving attention we place in setting the stage for ease each day. The magic in the space isn't technically the space; it's what happens there.

The rest of this chapter is dedicated to the steps you can take to create a comfortable environment of ease for your guest. Follow this advice and you'll be in a great position to begin your class with calm, happy people who've had a fantastic experience entering your space.

ARRIVE EARLY AND STAY LATE

You can't do much if you breeze into class a minute before it begins and hightail it out the moment it's over. If that's your style, you're giving the impression that you don't care much about the people in your class—you're telling them that you have somewhere better to be before and after. It's a bad habit to let yourself slip into, and it leaves you little chance of making a good impression or building a regular base of people who love what you lead.

Even if you're working at a place that has back-to-back classes, you can position yourself by the door before class begins and ends to greet people and answer questions. Before class you can offer to help people get situated. After class you can thank them for coming and answer any questions that may have come up. There is always a way to work with whatever you've got. Just like the practice. Ideally, it's good to arrive 20 to 30 minutes before your class begins to see what you can do to improve the environment and greet people as they arrive.

RESPECTFULLY CREATE THE ENVIRONMENT

Part of arriving early is about creating an environment of ease even before people get there.

When I travel and lead at other studios, conference centers, and open spaces, I arrive even earlier than I would for the classes at Strala NYC because usually there is more work to do. It's very important to me that I clean any space, set up mats evenly, and unclutter the environment wherever I am. Often at conferences I'm turning the room around to face the natural light, checking the sound system, putting on a playlist of welcoming and joyful music, and adjusting any lighting options I have. While a gym or hotel conference center may not seem like the ideal place to practice, it's possible to create a good feeling environment no matter where you are. Just show up early, clear the space, and set the stage for ease.

Every space is completely different, and there is a way to improve any space to create a more optimal environment. Even if the space isn't yours—if it's a shared or temporary space—there is a lot you can do without moving walls. As I've already mentioned, picking up clutter and trash and making sure the floor is swept go a long way. This attention to the space will also be positively noticed by the studio or club owner. Presenting yourself as someone who cares and improves conditions in your workplace is simply a sensible way to behave. Guides who don't care that there are a few empty cups or blankets left on the floor before their class begins aren't showing respect for the people coming to their classes. The same goes for not picking up the space afterward. This Guide isn't one I'd want to spend much time around, let alone employ.

Think of yourself as an entrepreneur whether you are the owner of the space or not. The more you can put yourself in the position of solving problems and improving things, the more valuable you are to yourself, those who come for your class, and potential employers and collaborators. If you have rigid ideas that you come only to teach and leave, you'll probably be replaced by the next Guide who comes in with a better attitude.

Another benefit to taking ownership of caring for the space is that this attitude rubs off. When I lead at the same studio for a while, or during a longer training with a group, the ethos of the group begins to change. People begin to pick up after themselves, respecting the space and others more. It feels good to live sustainably and show by example. By paying so much attention to the space, we notice that we are actually more connected to it than we can imagine. Our relationship with our surroundings is critical to our health. The physical room as our immediate environment becomes a practice ground for all our environments and our relationship to how we treat our planet. How much waste are we producing daily? Do we refill our water or use disposable cups? Do we pick up the trash, or do we treat the world as our garbage can? Sweeping the floor is a healing meditation. I do it daily.

It's important to me that if I'm leading a class, I'm the one to set up the space. It's not the job of whoever owns the gym or the cleaning people. Take responsibility for what you see and improve things for the experience as you respect the rules and guidelines of the space. No one is going to be upset if you sweep a floor or pick up a tissue. It's essential to take care of the space to create an environment of ease.

TEMPERATURE, LIGHT, SMELL & NOISE

How cold or warm is your space? Is there a good amount of natural light or overhead lighting? What does it smell like? Are there any unwanted noises that could be disruptive? Dealing with any problems in these areas is another reason it's good to arrive early. Leave ample time to make adjustments to the temperature, light, smell, and noise.

If the space is too cold, are there heaters that can be turned on? If it's too hot, are there windows or fans that can be opened and turned on? Are the fans in a good place to ventilate the room? Are they too noisy to have on during class, and maybe best used only before people show up? Do you need to air out the room before guests arrive?

Handling the lighting is also critical. Get to know where the light switches are and if there are dimmers. Think about which way makes sense for your class to face. Are there windows and natural light? If not, how can you make the best environment possible with the lighting options you have.

Smells—good or bad—can be utterly distracting when you practice. Are there musty or perfume smells in the room? Can you smell food? Is there anything that might give people a headache? Running the fans for a bit is a habit we are in before and after classes to bring the room back to a neutral smell. In the case of a studio, neutral is definitely the best.

Are there distracting noises in the building or in the room? It's good to come early in case there are. This leaves you with time to do some investigating so you can do something about it.

I was in London recently to lead a two-week training, and the space I rented presented several challenges. It had looked great on the website that advertised it, but when I arrived two days before the training started, I realized that it needed a lot of work. It's a good thing we were there early, because there were major things that needed attention.

The first emergency was the massive construction happening directly down-stairs. The drilling sounded like King Kong invading the building, so we talked to the guys who'd rented us the space. Since they threw their hands up and weren't much help, we decided to talk to the construction workers themselves. It obviously wasn't their fault that there was so much noise. The people who'd rented us the space really should have warned us about it—if they had, we wouldn't have rented it. So we talked with the construction guys nicely, explaining our situation, and they worked with us. They agreed to do their loud drilling during our lunch breaks and at night when our sessions were over. The noise was an ongoing situation during the weeks, but building that relationship with the construction workers was critical to solving the problem. Most of the people in the training group said hello to the guys on a daily basis. We had found a harmony that worked for both of us to do what we needed to do.

The space was also quite a bit smaller than advertised, and it was filled with tables, clutter, and decorations. I wanted the space to be as open, clear, and as free of decorations as possible. This would help people have a spacious and internal experience—not one focused on the decor. Thankfully I was able to clear the clutter and create a practice room. I arrived an hour early each day to make sure the noise situation was under control and to make sure the heat was fully on.

By the end of the program, my job was easier because everyone started to pitch in, picking up their cups and mats, organizing the room, and taking care of what we had. It was natural and a lovely feeling of camaraderie that created quite a bond between us and also with the space, as if it was our yoga home that we took such nice care of. We even cleaned up and swept on the last night and locked up our temporary home with love.

Being able to navigate through the unexpected frustrations in life is one of the reasons we do this practice. The attitude of calmly handling the noise and the mess is the same attitude we have with ourselves on the mat. How we practice is how we live, so it's vital to practice how we want to live all the time, whether the situation is easy or challenging. Challenges present even more opportunity for growth.

TUNES

Music is a topic I love to dive into because it's an incredibly powerful tool for setting the mood and supporting the class experience. I have several different before- and after-class playlists to create the appropriate atmosphere for each class. Just like everything else we've been discussing, music matters a whole lot. It's not just about putting on an upbeat group of songs before an ENERGIZE class to pump everyone up, or playing the chill tunes to relax everyone before a GENTLE or RELAX class; it's about carefully considering the circumstances and deciding how to support the experience you're aiming to give.

If you're going to use music, and I suggest that you do in most situations, it's crucial to get really interested in music, and not just the artists you listen to on the weekends with your friends. Music creates the atmosphere and speaks on a subconscious level to how we feel. Because of music's ability to tap into the subconscious, we must consider what we subject people to in the class environment.

Music is a super way to have natural interaction with those who come to your class. It's a natural connection. People love an inspirational playlist that got them through those handstand rocks attempts, or supported them on their boat ride, or helped them feel so at ease in pigeon. We Guides share our playlists with one another all the time. This helps us discover new music, get suggestions, and talk about feedback from people in the classes. If you're new to creating a before-, after-, or during-class playlist, we've got you covered until you start to incorporate the music that feels most natural to you. Check out our Spotify channel for some inspiration. You can access it from the social bar at the top of www.stralayoga.com.

When we discuss music in training groups, we often talk about "yoga music" versus "contemporary music" in regard to what is appropriate and effective for our classes. From our point of view, we aim to help people connect to themselves, so any music that supports that connection is appropriately called "yoga music." Often what we acknowledge as traditional yoga music gives the feeling that yoga has to do with something outside our current culture and day-to-day lives, and even outside ourselves. But that's not what Strala Yoga is about. It's about you in your life every day. It's internal. So we don't want people to get the impression they have to listen to something they would never listen to otherwise. The music shouldn't feel like it's from some other dimension, time, or place.

This doesn't mean, however, that we have to listen to the Top 40 hits of today. In fact, a playlist composed of only these songs creates a pretty flat experience. There are lovely songs and artists, like Krishna Das, that have a present-day resonating sound while singing some literal yoga-themed music. Creating playlists with a healthy variety of genres that embody a supportive, uplifting, and positive vibe is what gives your class a well-rounded experience full of the feeling of space and possibilities.

Whatever music you play, consider how it affects the people in your class—not just you. If you exclusively play your favorite artists, you likely need to expand your repertoire. Look at each song you consider and ask yourself how it makes you feel. Then ask yourself how it might make a group feel. The answers to these two questions might be extraordinarily different. A heavy metal fan and a jazz fan would definitely have different reactions to songs. Try to choose songs that won't offend people—even if they are outside their normal genres.

If you want to prepare a special music-inspired class for an event, like classical, hip-hop, or disco night, that can be really enjoyable for people, but it's best to prepare them in advance by advertising this aspect. Don't spring your love of the Bee Gees on people without warning.

So for each playlist you put together, ask yourself these questions: Is the effect of the music aligned with the goal of my class? Does the music ignite a connection with the people in my class?

Here are four factors to keep in mind when choosing your welcome and post-class playlists, as well as your in-class playlists.

1. FEELING: This is your gut reaction. What does the song feel like? Is it pleasing, soothing, energetic, or full of anxiety, sadness, or joy? We want to avoid songs that simmer in sadness or are full of rage. Although it's quite natural for someone to experience sadness in a class at some point, we choose not to enhance that sadness with sad music. We choose songs that are uplifting, energetic, soft, full of energy, and generally supportive of positivity. That's not a suggestion to fill your playlists with cartoon theme songs but to be mindful of how the songs feel. Consider the lyrics and the voice if there is a singer. What is the message of the song, and how does the singer's voice feel? Is it uplifting, energetic, and supportive? If so, then it might be a candidate.

2. VARIETY: Are your playlists full of your favorite artists, or do they have a wide variety of music? Are you subjecting everyone in the room to your devotion to the artist you've idolized since age 10, or are your choices more inclusive and well rounded, welcoming many ages, backgrounds, and types of people to your classes? Beware that if you choose to play only the music you love, you'll narrow your audience to a small group that thinks, acts, looks, and dresses just like you. If you broaden your selections and expand your choices, you'll widen your groups in diversity, interests, and vibrancy.

When it comes to changing your playlist, we suggest feathering in new songs every so often. Use your common sense to know when it's time for a shift in energy. Changing two or three songs at a time is enough to have a dramatic effect of newness. Changing too many songs at once has the risk of lost familiarity. People can get quite connected to your music if you do a good job of picking it out. A good playlist will make people feel supported, welcomed, and engaged. So stay interested and observe reactions to songs; then use your experience and intuition to guide you.

3. SUPPORT OF MOVEMENT WAVES: We'll get into "waves" in Chapter 8, but as you're putting together your playlist, consider what part of the class is happening and what music you are playing for that particular part. You'll soon learn that we structure classes with waves of movement to accomplish certain things. Having the music support the feeling of the movement we're creating helps people practice. Many classes begin with a lower-intensity practice, then move to something more difficult before chilling out again. If that's the case, your music should do the same thing. Like one big wave starting low with a steady rise and softly settling back down. A fantastic playlist makes sense as its own wave, as one cohesive, supportive experience.

Outside the actual class, music is a great tool for setting or changing the vibe in the room. I recently led a handstand workshop that ended not long before a RELAX class was about to begin. As the handstand workshop finished, the energy in the room was big and fun. I needed to do something to change the energy to be ready to relax. As the handstand group lingered around practicing their movements, even after class was over, I changed the playlist from the upbeat post-class celebratory music, which added a nice climax to the "we just did handstands!" workshop, to soft, ambient music so the relax group coming in would be welcomed into a calm space. It was a risk, but it worked like a charm. The happy handstanders started to wind down gently, collected themselves, and either settled in for RELAX class or headed back out into the world. The RELAX group started to come in and felt welcomed into a safe and serene environment. If I had chosen to keep the celebratory music on, the handstanders might have been motivated to handstand all the way until the moment the RELAX class started, and the group entering might have felt left out and wondering about all this chaos in the studio. A playlist goes a long way when you use it mindfully.

4. VOLUME: While this may seem obvious, volume is something I feel I need to address—because it is incredibly important. You don't want to struggle to be heard because you have the volume on your music up too high. You also don't want to have it so low that it's not able to support the experience fully. A nice volume is one that fills the room with sound, while being quiet enough that you can hear the conversations with people as they come in. This pre-class assessment will likely help you figure out a good volume so people can hear your instructions.

If you are using a remote to control volume, make it part of your body and your movement in a way. Be graceful with the remote. Find a way to set it down gently when you aren't using it, or tuck it in your shirt if it's tiny. Use the remote as another tool and element in your guiding. Raising the volume a bit during moments of free moving and breathing time can be supportive of the experience. Softening the volume when you are leading and in final relaxation is equally supportive and powerful.

Whether using a remote or not, choosing a volume that supports the experience, one you and your class don't feel challenged by, is critical to feeling at ease. Music can be that extra element that helps people do more with less effort. Use it as a tool, and you'll enjoy the success it can deliver.

Music brings joy, and putting together music for others brings loads of joy. I encourage you to listen to a lot of music, create lots of playlists, and do your practice to them to see how they feel. Practice by yourself and with your friends many times before you take the music to the studio or club. Just like everything else, becoming the master of music as a tool for the experience comes with experience. The more you dive into listening to all kinds of music and putting together those playlists—and watching how they affect people in your classes—the more you'll understand firsthand the power of music to support the environment. This is the fun stuff, so enjoy it.

WRAPPING IT UP

Everything about setting up your studio and getting the word out should be enjoyable. It should stir up a sense of excitement in you. It should focus on connecting with others. You're captaining the ship, conducting the orchestra, welcoming people into your class, and presenting them with a wonderful healing experience of ease.

The basic idea with everything I've suggested is that you create your space as you would if the person you most respected in the world was about to come over and experience it. If you do this, you'll bring out the most wonderful qualities in your guests.

The most crucial concept to remember is that all this is living, breathing, and evolving, and you improve immensely with practice. No two classes will ever be the same. No two people entering your space will be the same. No two spaces you lead in will be the same. What an exciting opportunity to learn how to thrive in any situation. This is the practice of sharpening your skills at evolution! If you are interested in leading, I encourage you to consider your attitude, space, welcoming style, smell, and music for each class you lead. Get in there, see what improvements you can make, and when in doubt, breathe, soften, and move from your middle. How the space feels begins and ends with how you feel. Clearing the clutter, sweeping the floor, and choosing the music are the details; you will always be the most important element to your leading. This is great news since we always have complete control over ourselves and always have endless opportunities for improvement and lasting change.

Attitude is everything. Aim to be excellent, and your faults will shatter your ground. Aim to improve, and you will be excellent.

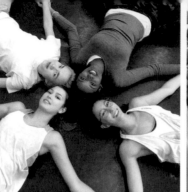
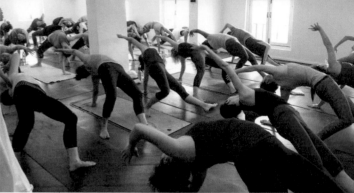
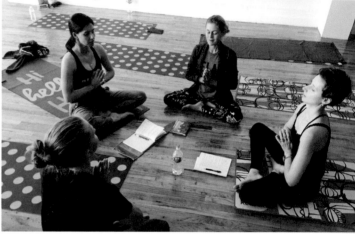
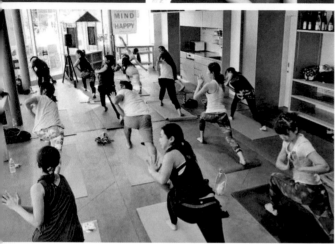

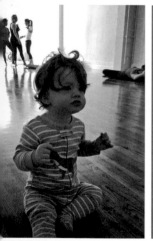
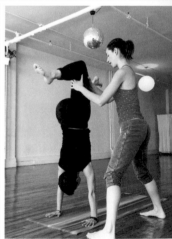

> " Forming a positive connection with others begins by forming a positive connection with yourself. "

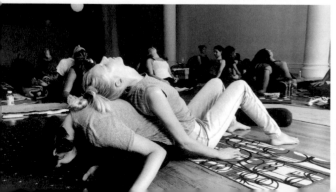
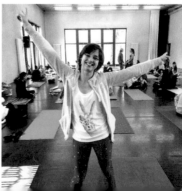

GUIDING MOVEMENT

MASTERING PHILOSOPHY, LANGUAGE & TOUCH

With your space set up and your attitude on the right track, it's time to get down to the business of learning how to actually guide a class. Leading class is like telling a story. It's the story of the breath, the story of the wave, the story of the heart and the connection we all share. It's always the same story, told in endless variations, experienced uniquely by countless individuals. This story comes to life in the energy of the Guide. You are the storyteller, involving your moving, living, breathing parts and all the people who show up to participate. You enjoy the honor of telling the story and being in the story as you soak it up with your listeners, who are also participants. They are your cast members. The breath is the star. The heart is the mysterious love interest, unable to be caught but pulled and pushed by the breath and the body. The theme is vast, deep, rich, heavy, light, comedic, and dramatic all at once. How you are will be the story you tell.

This is the core principle of guiding: the best way to guide is by example. But there are some specific techniques we focus on to create the feeling of ease and space that are part of the Strala experience.

Strala acknowledges physical, mental, emotional, and spiritual connection through clear and straightforward guiding of the process of expansive movement. We guide elegant simplicity through frame-by-frame instruction, allowing space for people to experience their own inner world, without layering on emotional or feeling-based language. In short, we strategically guide people through a process of exploration rather than telling them how to move and what to feel. The goal is for people to tap into their own body's knowledge to do what will be most beneficial for them.

simple leading concepts

* Clear straightforward language of frame-by-frame instruction

* Soft, easygoing movement with no end points

* Quality of movement, natural leading from the breath and belly

* Calm ease carried through easy and challenging moments alike

* Exploration into you, with no one correct way

* Focus on the process instead of an end point pose goal

* Emphasis on how I can help over what I can prove

* Priority on support and sensitization instead of a more contorted expression

* Complete start-to-finish experience

* Building strength and a healthy range of mobility with grace

* Movement phrases designed to feel expansive

* Soft, meditative movement

* Accomplishing challenging movements with ease

* Focused attention on the process to move beyond any one goal

THE LANGUAGE OF STRALA

So, how do we guide people without telling them what to do? This is a fine line that we constantly have to walk—we want to protect people from moving in ways that will hurt them yet leave things open enough to inspire exploration and introspection.

We guide actions instead of feelings. Saying, "Take a few moments to explore" is quite different from saying, "Take a few moments to feel the stretch in your legs, the length in your torso." In one, we're opening up the opportunity to tap into what the body is saying. In the other, we're telling people to notice specific things, which means that they aren't looking anywhere else. They are not truly exploring; they're just noticing. Guiding the feeling removes the participant from the experience. It also puts in place a strange power play—the Guide is in charge and the person in class is simply following directions. Instead we want to set up a solid container of movement and then let the feelings happen.

The clearer you are in guiding the actions, the more profound the feelings will be. The less you guide the feelings, the more individualized and beneficial the experience will be. Let your language be clear, concise, and confident.

ECONOMY OF WORDS

In an effort to create clear language that will help people feel into themselves, we need to look at how we talk about movement. The most simple and clear language you can use to guide and support the feeling of the movement enriches the experience and effectiveness of your leading. I recommend you use as few words as possible to describe the frame-by-frame action. Flowery, indulgent language pulls people out of the experience of themselves. At best, it connects the class to *your* feelings. At worst, it completely turns someone off, distracting them from their own feelings, which could lead to injury. Even if a person loves the flowery language you're using, you are simply entertaining them—you're not helping them go further inside to get the best results.

Simplicity of instructions connects the individual inward, to an endless expanse. Aim to be gracefully simple.

So let's look at a couple of examples to see what I'm talking about. This first one—although a bit exaggerated—shows just how distracting flowery language can be.

> Stand tall like you would if you just won a prize. Imagine the prize in your mind. It's yours. Take a big inhale, reach your arms up, and claim your prize. Okay, now we're gonna exhale and fold forward. Take the prize home. Bend your knees and step back to your low lunge. Get into your hips—imagine salsa dancing. Those hips can sway, slide, shimmy. But the hips hold a lot of the junk of our emotions, so you may start feeling uncomfortable as you move. Don't be afraid to work through any pain. It's probably your childhood coming up. Let it go.

I think that was pretty obviously bad. Let's look at an example of the same movement phrase, guided simply and clearly.

> Stand tall. Soften your knees, close your eyes, and draw your attention inward. Settle here for a moment. When you're ready, take a big inhale and reach your arms out and up. Exhale and soften over your legs. Soften your knees, shift your weight onto your right foot, and step your left foot back to your low lunge. Sink your hips here and sway a bit side to side if that feels nice.

As you can see, the experience of these two ways of talking about movement are exquisitely different. In the first one, the Guide was putting on a show. In the second, the Guide is trying to help you connect to you.

Another thing to keep in mind is to watch out for unnecessary phrases that do nothing other than waste time, energy, and breath. Here are some of the most commonly used wasteful guiding phrases to avoid:

* ❋ We're/You're gonna . . .
* ❋ Next . . .
* ❋ Now . . .
* ❋ On your next inhale/exhale . . .

These phrases are time wasters. They act to announce something you're going to lead before you lead it. For example: "We're gonna come into down dog split. Take a big inhale and lift your right leg into down dog split."

Get rid of the announcement phrase. Simply say, "Take a big inhale and lift your right leg into down dog split."

Instead of "On your next inhale, lift your arms over your head," use "Inhale your arms up over your head."

Another thing that muddies up language is using inclusive modifiers, such as *our* or *we*. For clarity, use *your*. This is the most efficient way to guide movement. Say both of these out loud:

❋ **Let's all inhale and lift our arms up overhead. Then we can exhale and bring our hands to center, thumbs to our heartbeat.**

❋ **Take a big inhale and lift your arms up overhead. Exhale and press your thumbs to your heartbeat.**

It may seem like a small, silly thing, but in the first example, you're asking a group to believe that we have one collective heartbeat.

Some people may argue that using *our* and *we* makes the experience more inclusive—that it creates more of a collective experience of movement. But from my experience with groups, the use of these terms simply distracts. So in Strala we aim to guide the person and let the group experience happen naturally.

The "our/we" language can come across childish. "Let's all lift our left leg up" can come across as babying the group, instead of "take a big inhale and lift your left leg up."

The lesson is to keep your instructions wonderfully simple, directed at connecting people inward to their own stories. This practice frees you to put your attention on the people in the room and support them in their exploration. When you are focused on your own story of emotion and feeling, there is no space for people to have any experience other than yours. How exhausting for you to take on all that weight. Drop the performance, put your attention on helping the people around you—because there will always be someone who needs help. In Chapter 8, we talk about some specific ways to guide breath, feeling, and natural movement, but keeping this general philosophy of language in mind—in all aspects of guiding—will take you in the right direction.

THE POWER OF VOICE

Along with avoiding the pretension of flowery language comes avoiding what I call "yoga voice." Something funny can happen when people get up in front of a room to lead yoga. They chat like a normal person before class, but then, when everyone calms down and gets ready to begin, their voice changes. As an experienced yoga practitioner, I imagine you've run into this once or twice. Yoga voice is characterized by an unnatural tone and pitch, and it's laced with the suggestion that this person is about to bestow a precious and spiritual gift on the people in class. By moving into this inauthentic "knowing" voice, the guide takes herself into the realm of teacher rather than Guide. Yoga voice implies that this person knows best. It implies that students should listen to the teacher.

The more you can simply be yourself when you're guiding, the more relatable you'll be and the easier it will be for the class to connect with themselves. So keep it natural and easy. Your real voice will work just fine. In fact, it will work better.

I don't want you to get so obsessed with keeping your voice authentic, however, that you go to the other end of the spectrum: speaking in monotone. Your voice should support the instruction. It should follow movement naturally in its tone and inflection. Let's give it a try. Say these two phrases without inflection as you move from warrior 2 to warrior 2 lift:

❋ Take a big inhale and lift your hips and arms up.

❋ Easy exhale and soften back to warrior 2.

Now put a bit of inflection in the instruction. In the first, your voice should carry a quality of lift. In the second, it should have a quality of softening and settling. Can you feel the difference when you allow your voice to be free so it can move with the movement?

If you speak the same tone the whole class, the experience feels flat and unsupported. The proper inflection in your natural voice can create a supportive, safe, expansive environment.

BODY POSITION, DEMONSTRATION & CONTACT

Where you are when you are leading is important. It's a great general rule to be where people can hear and see you. We start each class facing people in the center, mirroring and demonstrating the three breaths. When the class starts to move, the Guide immerses herself in the room to make contact with people.

Figuring out where to be during the class is tough. We've all experienced someone standing too close or not close enough—and the proximity problem really makes things uncomfortable. Unfortunately, what is the correct distance has no simple answer. It's something that you will figure out as you lead. With practice you'll hone your awareness of what makes sense. You will learn to quickly feel what will be most effective.

I'll admit I've had countless experiences where I made contact with someone that was awkward. I was a little too close or a little too far. But through the years, I've improved. It's all in experience. This is one of the areas where

I recommend you bring in your friends for practice. Guide them through a class. Experiment. And then ask for useful, critical feedback. Encourage your practice partners to be honest and specific. Not just "that felt nice" or "that wasn't so great." You're looking for feedback like, "It would have been nice if you were a little closer during that downward dog" or "I couldn't hear you when we were moving through that sun salutation because you were too far away."

Specifics like this help you figure out what works and what doesn't. Oh, so much to play with.

Aside from figuring out proximity for personal comfort, you also need to figure out how best to move through the room so people get the most out of the experience. There are times when you stay in front of the class to demonstrate, but for most usual-size classes, say, a handful of people up to a full room in a studio, it's useful to spend some time moving through the room instead of parking yourself in the front for the entire class.

Moving through the room not only puts you in connection with each person; it creates a feeling of openness and ease. I recommend that as the Guide you don't use a mat. Part of the reasoning behind this is simply to remind you to move, but the other part is to keep people's focus on themselves. If you set up shop at the front of the room, doing every move you instruct, people's natural inclination will be to pay complete attention to you. If you move around the room, not demonstrating everything but rather guiding movement with your words, your voice, and your tone, people will pay attention to themselves.

How you move about—or *if* you move about—will change depending on the circumstances. Sometimes it's impossible to get out into the group. For example, you may be in a special situation, like leading a giant class with hundreds of people, where you are essentially glued to a stage so a camera can follow you. I had one large-scale event in Prague where I had to lead about 2,000 people through an entire class from a high platform, in a dark room with a light show going on and a spotlight on me. I couldn't see anyone, much less move into the crowd. I could barely see my own feet. It was one of the most challenging classes I've had to lead. I had no idea how it was going for everyone, or if I was going to fall off the platform if I lost my balance.

Luckily most of the time you won't be leading in the dark—figuratively or literally. Even in big group classes where guiding from a stage is an effective approach, you might still have a chance to hop off the stage when people are doing those exploratory movements, like handstand, pigeon, or final relaxation.

Each circumstance is unique, and when you gain experience, figuring out how to move about a class becomes effortless and easy. That's the fun of leading all kinds of classes. The more you lead, the more exposure you get to all kinds of crazy things happening. After years of leading, it will be almost impossible to throw you off your optimal guiding.

TO DEMONSTRATE OR NOT TO DEMONSTRATE

The decision of whether or not to demonstrate a movement is similar to the decision of where to be: it's different in every situation. Sometimes it makes sense to mirror every move, standing in front of the crowd. Sometimes it makes sense to only demonstrate at the very beginning. Sometimes guiding sporadically throughout the class is the way to go. It depends both on the setting and the type of class. If you're focusing on a group of people who are mostly beginners, demonstration is helpful, but even with this, you still want to get out around the room and interact with people.

MIRRORING & DIRECTIONS

When you are demonstrating, keep in mind where you are facing and how that affects the group being able to see, hear, and follow you clearly. Mirroring is the clearest way to demonstrate movement to a group. If you are new to mirroring, take the time to try it on and get familiar with it. Your right side becomes your left side and the other way around. Like anything new, it will take a lot of practice to be comfortable and master mirroring, but it is a powerful tool that helps you be able to see and connect with the group. People are able to follow the direction because you are moving like a mirror image. Let's look at the alternatives. If you stand facing away from the group, you are able to do the class with the group, but you can't see anyone, which makes helping impossible. If you stand facing parallel in front of the group, guiding movement to movement becomes confusing. When you turn from front to back while the group is turning from left to right, you cut off your vision half of the time also. In all forms of movement, from tai chi to dance, mirroring has been handed down through the generations. It works and is wonderful when you gain confidence in leading this way.

We also choose not to put a mat for the Guide in the front of the room, unless it's a special event and you're on a stage leading a giant group. As I said before, having no mat frees you up to move about the room and demonstrate your mirroring from the front middle, or slightly to one side or the other, depending on where the people are in your class. We usually place a folded blanket in the front of the room to organize the space. It's something we use to sit on in the beginning and the end of class and it orients the group by showing which way is front.

After assessing who's in a class, you can choose to go heavy on demonstrating or not. There is so much support you can provide when you're not doing the movements. Think about an orchestra. A conductor stands in front of the orchestra and clearly guides the action of the musicians without ever playing a note. The support he provides comes from body position, movements, and passionate and clear cuing.

When you're walking through the class, remember that your body can lift and soften like a wave and move gently and effortlessly like the wind. Your breath should be deep and full. Your tone and voice should be clear and natural. Using your voice and body as your instrument is exciting. These are all ways you can support without demonstrating.

You need to always stay aware of how your class is going. If people seem frustrated or lost, they will likely shut down. In these instances demonstrating can bring them back to the point of feeling. It may provide just the comfort needed for them to relax into exploration.

The beauty of Strala is that we help people connect to themselves—and putting the focus on the people in class facilitates this. If someone just wanted demonstration, they could watch a video at home. Moving out into the class helps you connect with people. To observe them and give them the personalized support they need. People come to a class for many reasons. Whether it's motivation of the group, connection and support from the Guide, or information on the process, it's our job to give them what they're looking for.

PHYSICAL TOUCH & SUPPORT

Part of giving people support is about making physical contact. This can be a touchy subject (pun intended!). Some people are comfortable being touched and others aren't. So your goal is to make contact and then allow space for a reaction. For most people, a gentle, helpful touch will inspire an adjustment that leads to increased comfort, ease, or healing. This happens in the reaction to the touch, not in the touch itself. We are not physically moving people with touch. We are inspiring adjustment by bringing attention to something. Our techniques come from the spirit of do no harm and the attitude of support instead of manipulate. We don't have to "do anything" or "fix someone" when we touch them, instead we apply techniques of relaxation and leaning to help the person find comfort and support in the movement.

Let's look at a few types of touch. The first is *informative*. An informative touch is simply a quick way to provide information to someone. For example, you could make contact in an informative way if someone is standing with their shoulders visibly tense. A direct and clear touch with your hands on their shoulders might help them soften. Remember, just like verbal leading, match what you say and what you do—be soft and relaxed when you are helping someone soften and relax.

A *supportive* touch is a wonderful way to help people connect with themselves and find their own best way into the movement. We often talk about supportive touch as "leaning" because you are literally leaning some of your body weight on someone else in a way where both of you are supported. This technique is the basis of many healing arts.

We don't have to dwell too much on the final type of touch here: inappropriate touch. Any touch that creates a superficial connection like petting, stroking, or massaging is inappropriate. But even an okay touch can feel inappropriate when it's approached with indecision, or from a place where the receiver isn't aware it is coming, or in a place where it's unwelcomed or not okay to touch in the context of a yoga class. We also want to avoid harsh mechanical manipulation.

UNDERSTANDING TOUCH

There is no one better to talk about the issue of touch than Strala faculty member Sam Berlind. Sam is a no-rules ninja, same as Mike, with incredibly disciplined and diverse experiences of training in touch and support, specifically shiatsu. During his studies of comparative religion and philosophy at the University of Edinburgh, Sam became curious about the practical aspects of his academic research, so he began to explore yoga and meditation. After moving to New York, he continued to practice and began to teach yoga, focusing on the relationship between the practice of yoga and traditional Asian healing arts. Sam studied Chinese herbal medicine, acupuncture, martial arts, and shiatsu with Pauline Sasaki and Wataru Ohashi. Learning about touch, movement, healing, and the relationship between them fascinated him, and he dived deeply into the field. He's taught all around the world, speaks several languages, and spends time with us in Strala and teaching touch in the training programs.

His approach to touch isn't strict shiatsu, which claims that each point that we make mechanical contact with affects the body and the energy in a certain way. Sam brings the integrity of shiatsu back, recognizing that healing happens not from the point of touch or the amount of pressure but in the response of the receiver. Sam's approach is about using our whole selves to connect with another person to provide the space for support and healing. We're going for an internal reaction, not an external reaction, such as one that would be the result of a massage. By learning an approach, instead of fixating on specific techniques, we understand and become effective in creating opportunity for this lasting change we hope to effect in those we connect with.

This section with Sam gives you a great approach to touch—he also gives you some exercises to try, so grab a partner.

SAM:

WHY TOUCH?

There are many good reasons to use touch when guiding a Strala class, but this is the most important: each time we touch or are touched creates an opportunity for change and growth. We touch to make a connection, to create a relationship with another person in a special way. Of course, everything you do with people creates the experience of connectedness: the way you use your voice and what you choose to say, how you move through the physical space of a studio, the way you demonstrate movement, the music and the lighting . . . but one of the most powerful tools we have is touch.

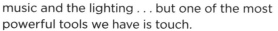

Tactile stimulation is a fundamentally necessary part of our early growth, one of our basic needs along with food, water, oxygen, rest, and activity. Touching our own body is often our first response to pain, stress, anxiety, or excitement. We *know* ourselves through touching and being touched, creating our sense of identity from our physical contact with the environment. "I feel, therefore I am": touching tells us where and who we are and gives us the feedback we need to make adjustments in our movement and behavior in order to change the patterns of our lives.

When you lean on someone, even for a few seconds, you are choosing to trust them to support you, and that in turn inspires them to trust you. It's in the relationship that you choose to create that an opportunity for change and healing happens. Trust is the basic technique we need for touching people; who, when, and where to touch, for how long, with how much of our body weight—these are refinements.

EXERCISE

Sit back to back with a partner, legs folded or extended, lean back and find the way to support each other with perfect ease. Breathe, relax, and feel how much your partner is "doing" while seeming to do nothing at all. Exchange feedback.

How did that feel? What did you notice about yourself? Were you also aware of your partner's breath or experience?

Touch is touch, whether with your back, a hand, a forearm, or a knee. We touch with our whole selves, from the center, not with a part.

DON'T FIX

Proper alignment, correct posture, avoiding injury, physical improvement, or achieving the perfect asana are often the stated goals of both yoga teachers and students.

When we "correct" the alignment or posture of someone through touch or word, we are implying that there are universal principles of yogic alignment that we know and should be teaching others. As if the goal of yoga practice is to achieve some kind of ideal symmetry or balance, as if a perfect pose awaits our mastery.

But how does it really work? Think of how we first learn to move as babies. It's not through instruction but by spontaneous experimenting, playing with movement, and finding the way that works best for us. A healthy child resists being helped. She wants to figure it out for herself. No one taught us how to reach for our mothers, to crawl, or to walk.

Do you, as a Guide, know more than other people about how they feel and function? Or about how, exactly, they should rotate a shoulder, angle a pelvis, or place a foot to move more easily and comfortably? Don't fix or educate people. Making appropriate contact with them gives them the information they need to teach themselves.

We are responsible for learning how to move our own bodies through playful exploration, how to create that sense of ease and pleasure in ourselves. Your responsibility is to be completely present and enjoy yourself while guiding the class. Graceful movement is showing, not telling, people how to move. Use touch to create a relationship in which you demonstrate how relaxed, trusting, and easy movement can feel.

EXERCISE

Have your partner lie facedown while you sit or squat comfortably nearby. Close your eyes, breathe in, and lean with one or both hands onto your prone partner. Your only purpose is to be supported. Open your eyes, switch places, and repeat. Exchange feedback.

Did you notice that the person leaning in "accidentally" chose the right place to touch? How did that happen? What part did trust play in this experiment?

Your touch is both supportive and challenging to the other person. They will react by feeling and understanding something about themselves, and this will inform their yoga practice. We are responsible for ourselves! An easy way to understand this is by thinking about what can happen when someone who cares for you offers you friendly advice. You appreciate their intention (to support you), consider their advice (which may feel challenging), and then decide for yourself how to act.

CHOOSING WHO, WHEN, WHERE & HOW TO TOUCH

We all have different ways of receiving information and understanding other people. Perhaps someone describes an injury or asks for help understanding a movement before or after class: through a dialogue with the other person, you reach a conclusion based on the data received. Or you might visually analyze their posture based on your experience and knowledge of anatomy and movement. This may require years of study and practice.

Alternatively, can use your gut instinct, allowing your intuition to guide your perception of the person and their situation. This is something we all know how to do; we recognize with a glance whom we trust, fear, or like. We almost instantly know who's expressing discomfort, sadness, or joy in their faces or postures.

We're all different: some of us feel more through touch, some listen to the tone and quality of other peoples' voices, some of us instinctively use our noses, and some of us are predominantly visual. We can develop each of these ways of knowing through practice.

Let's play with using our intuitive visual sense, a useful ability when guiding a roomful of people.

EXERCISE

Close your eyes and relax them for a moment, then open them as you exhale, taking in as much of the visual field as possible, not focusing on any object or individual, much less any details. Notice to whom and what your relaxed eyes are attracted, without analyzing the reason for this. Notice how it feels to be really *seen* by someone else.

Did you trust your first impression? Where was your attention pulled? Who or what was interesting to you? Try this 10 times, each time using your breath and choosing without hesitation, so that you begin to feel confident. You can play with this in almost any ordinary moment in your life with other people, especially strangers.

The end of class presents an easy opportunity to practice touch: the students are usually relaxed, receptive, and unlikely to interpret your touch as corrective. Any place from the knees down is generally perceived as nonthreatening and safe. Contact with the shoulders or neck is fine; bear in mind that we are more protective of our upper bodies, necks, and faces, so your approach should be especially graceful. Whatever you choose, be gentle yet decisive. Massaging, rubbing, and tentative movements don't create the same deep relationship that leaning with trust does.

EXERCISE

One person in final relaxation pose, the other 10 feet away. Look with relaxed eyes, be pulled to any place from the knees down, exhale, lean, and support. Take three slow breaths and then, with an exhalation, lean away from your partner (and resume guiding your imaginary class). Switch, exchange feedback.

Try this several times with different partners, each time finding an easier way of making the transition from touching to not touching. Invite your partners to be direct in their feedback—they are your best teachers.

Use relaxed eyes to observe a "student" in supine position, choose whether to contact upper (neck, shoulders) or lower body, approach, make contact. Ask for feedback, "How did that feel? Did I choose the right place to touch?" Switch roles.

The precise target you choose for your palms or thumbs matters less than the feeling you make contact with. Trust your ability to choose and then commit yourself. You can experiment with choosing particular acupressure/shiatsu points or simply let intuition guide your hands.

When touching students during standing poses, be sure not to unbalance them: move close to them and then use your entire body through your hands to make contact. As you practice and feel more confident, you'll invent your own ways to support/challenge your students.

───────────── EXERCISE ─────────────

Form small groups and role-play, creating different ways to understand and touch in a variety of poses. Start with child's pose, pigeon, seated forward bends, and twists and then move to standing, balancing positions.

When in the role of student, tell the Guide what you need in terms of touch, what feels wonderful, not so wonderful. Using phrases like "I am feeling . . ." and "I would like you to . . ." is a great way to communicate with others without correcting or teaching them.

TOUCH APPROPRIATELY

You already know how to observe and establish appropriate boundaries with other people. Avoid body contact that is rough, forceful, or unnecessarily intimate (for example, don't press your pelvis against someone's hip in a forward bend). More important, when in the role of Guide, be clear about your intentions with people, not manipulative or seductive.

"WHAT DO I DO WITH MY HANDS? WHAT AM I SUPPOSED TO BE FEELING?"

Don't worry about how to use your hands: relax, use them naturally, and feel with your entire being/body. Feeling is not a mysterious, elusive skill; we do it all the time in every life activity. Breathe and you will become confident and natural in the way you use touch in your yoga classes.

Use your entire body to do any simple, repetitive movement at home, vacuuming, washing dishes, cutting vegetables, and so on, hands relaxed to the point of almost dropping things, moving from your center. Notice how effortless every task becomes.

WHEN TO AVOID TOUCH

While most people will be helped by a gentle touch, some people want to be left alone. If they ask you not to by word or strongly imply it with body language (for example, arms or legs crossed, eyes wide-open in final relaxation pose), don't touch them.

If someone always asks you for touch, make sure to not give preferential treatment. Other people need your attention too.

If someone appears extremely emotionally volatile, unstable, or drugged, don't touch. A class is a shared group situation, not a therapy session, and we want to avoid

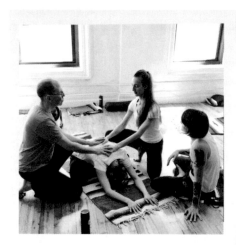

provoking a reaction that may require special, private attention.

And remember, you're important too. If you really don't want to touch someone, don't!

Most yoga studios work under an assumption of implied consent, meaning that students implicitly agree and understand that the teacher may touch them in a class. But if you are in doubt, just ask.

Touch can be a very powerful tool if you use it correctly. You can help people avoid injuries by using a gentle, leaning touch instead of correcting with forceful pushing and pulling. Encourage and support—don't teach. A thoughtful touch can inspire others to make the small or large adjustments necessary to find the right balance between mobility and stability in their practice. Demonstrate with your presence, movement, and touch what it feels like to move easily and without unnecessary effort.

OPPORTUNITIES FOR CONTACT

Sam talked a bit about times in class when touch can make a huge difference. There are also some of the other sensible places where we can make physical contact in class. Let's go over a few of them here. Grab a partner, and don't forget to ask them for critical feedback. The pickier your partner is on the quality of the touch, the more you'll learn and improve.

HANDSTAND

Handstands are a wonderful opportunity to get to know yourself. It's not the handstand that is so incredible, but it's what happens to our minds when we turn ourselves upside down and support ourselves in a new way that is remarkable. We offer a support that provides the most choice and freedom for our partner and is easy and safe for us to accomplish.

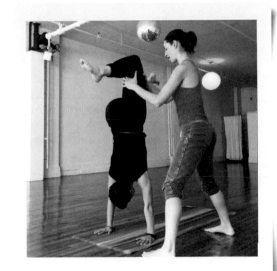

Before we make contact we want to make sure we are relaxed and easy. We have a wide, athletic stance, and soft joints. We are ready. We stand beside the person, on the side of the leg that they are lifting. The lifting leg is the one we will support. Placing a hand on the top of their thigh (will be closer to the ground) and the other hand on the bottom of their thigh (will be facing up) grab hold firmly, soften your knees, and move with them as they lift up into handstand. By having one leg supported, the person has freedom to move as they wish and come down as they wish. If he bends his elbows and melts to a dangerous position, you can easily lift him up and bring him down to safety. If she uses too much or not enough force to lift up, you can stabilize her with this support. Get to know many different partners in this movement so you are prepared if you choose to guide handstand and know that everyone moves and responds differently. Our main aim is to be there to support and provide safety.

DOWN DOG

Down dog is another easy place to make a connection. Although there are many places you could touch someone, grab someone, lift and adjust someone, remember we are here to support and not manipulate bodies. It can be tempting,

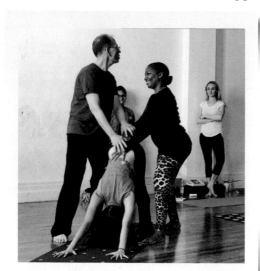

depending on your background, to want to get someone into a deeper expression of the pose, but it's important to remember we aren't here to correct and manipulate an external shape. The goal is an internal reaction.

Starting from a comfortable, easy position, bring your whole self as you approach your partner. It will probably make the most sense to come from the side and make contact with the lower or middle back. If you notice your partner's head is tense or hamstrings are tight, making contact with the lower or middle back will inform them to soften and relax. They will probably adjust, bend their knees a bit, and relax a bit more. We are going for the middle of the body here, not moving end points such as moving a head to a different position or pressing heels toward the floor. It's wonderful what is possible when you provide support at the center and allow the body to ripple and relax from the middle on out.

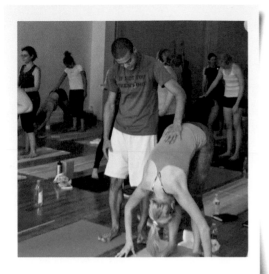

STANDING FORWARD BEND

The same principles apply here as always. Again, come from the side to make contact at the lower or middle back. I note that you should come from the side because if you stand behind or in front of someone in a forward bend, it's hard not to tip them over, even with the most careful touch.

PIGEON

For pigeon, as with every movement, take in the whole person. Knee safety is often an issue in this pose. We wouldn't want to lean on someone whose hips are way up and who looks as if she is balancing on her knee for support. A nice support for someone who is uncomfortable in pigeon is coming alongside him, getting into the pigeon yourself, and helping him explore around the movement to find a place where he feels a good opening but can still breathe easily and fully. From a comfortable place, it might be appropriate to connect with touch. A hand or forearm on the back and a gentle lean might be a nice support. Every person and every situation is different, so make sure not to one-size-fits-all for each position.

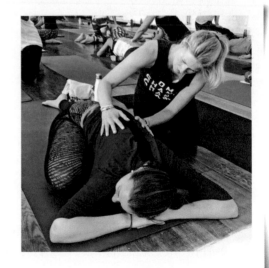

CHILD'S POSE

The same kind of knee safety applies for child's pose. Although it's a position some people love, it is quite uncomfortable for others. Leaning on someone when they are uncomfortable or their knees are challenged is not

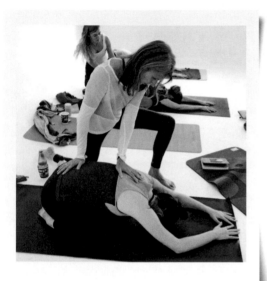

good, and could injure the person physically as well as provide emotional discomfort and stress. Make sure to take in the whole person before you approach. Often the right application of touch is to leave the person alone. If you see the person is comfortable and decide to approach, try getting on the same level, coming down to a squat position or kneeling so you are mobile and relaxed, and make contact from there.

PRACTICE, PRACTICE, PRACTICE

When it comes to making contact, we can never get enough practice. Continue to lean on each other, lean on your partner, try things, experiment, and ask for critical feedback. You won't have the opportunity to ask for feedback in your classes, so continue to practice on your friends, family, yoga partners, and peers. Allow yourself to be a beginner. The biggest mistake you could make is rushing through, considering this area of learning accomplished and checked off, and not continuing to play around and explore. It's a forever journey that you'll get better at with time. If it's comfortable, fun, and easy now, great; keep practicing. If it's awkward, uncomfortable, and challenging, that's okay too; keep practicing.

I've been leaning on people in yoga classes as a Guide for more than a decade and I improve month to month, year to year. Mike has been doing this for several years longer than me. Sam has been doing this for more than 30 years, so he has some experience on us. It's not just the passage of time that helps you improve. It's the dedication and regular practice plus the time that leads to gaining more confidence and developing a clear sense of what works with different people. Take an interest in people. Take an interest in people's posture, how they are, what they say, how they hold themselves, and see if you can keep the whole person in mind when you connect. Put yourself in service and focus on improving your skills, and you will always have a great class.

It's incredible the average shelf life for a body worker is just a few years. Most people burn out, become injured, or feel emotionally drained from giving so much to the people they are helping. With a more balanced approach to healing, touch, support, and listening, the Guide is actually being supported. You end up feeling great when you are supporting others. I want to be able to Guide for my whole life, and I'm grateful that this approach energizes and inspires. We are replenishing ourselves when we guide and connect with others. It's freeing to not take the perspective of advising, fixing, and correcting everyone. Offering support feels great for both parties and is effective, just like the warm hug of your friend when you are in need.

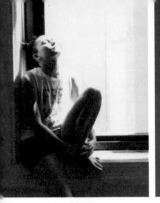
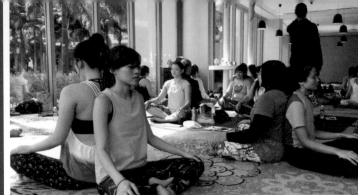
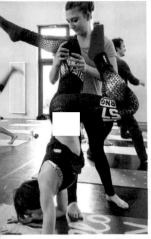

> "
> When you lead people, give them room to move, freedom, and a structure for progress.
> "

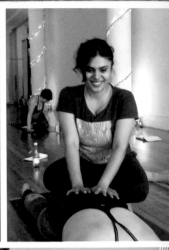
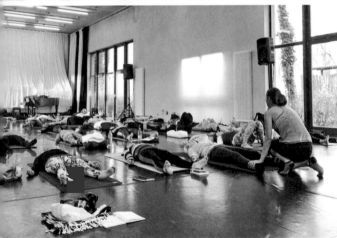
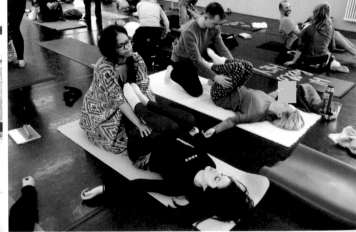
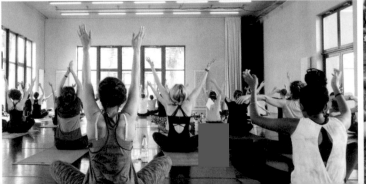
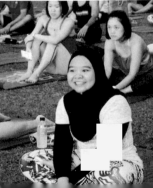

chapter
8

WAVES & FLOW

GUIDING BREATH, FEELING & STRUCTURING A CLASS

Now for the really fun stuff! Let's get into the specifics of guiding the three pieces of the Strala philosophy: breath, feeling, and natural movement.

GUIDING BREATH

There's a lot more to cuing the breath than simply repeating "inhale" and "exhale" before every movement instruction. While you do instruct this sometimes, the most important part of guiding people to their breath is your own breathing! By creating a breath-body connection for yourself, you help others do the same.

The breath-body connection and movements of the Guide actually create a huge part of the experience of the class. You should use your own breath to initiate a lift of your body each time you instruct an inhale. You should soften yourself as you instruct an exhale. While you may not be demonstrating the movement itself, you are creating the same feeling of lift that you hope to inspire in others. Obviously you can't actually breathe in while you guide the inhale. It's simply not possible to breathe in as you speak, but you can feel the lift in your body. Same with the exhale. Feel the softening of your body. Your breathing will happen naturally in moments when you aren't speaking.

When demonstrating movement, the same principles apply. Breathing comes first. Without the breath, instruction is just movement with the feeling removed. Without the feeling, the connection to the self and the ability to sensitize, relax, restore, and accomplish more with less effort vanishes. The breath is the beginning and continuation of everything. This is why a Guide who breathes deeply is essential to creating a supportive environment and informative instruction. This focus on leading the breath by example helps the people in class relax and breathe more deeply themselves. So take big, deep breaths consistently as you guide, and you'll find the natural rhythm.

The reason a class feels good is because the Guide is relaxed, at ease, and applying principles of soft, efficient movement, fueled by the breath. When they lead from a place of breathing deeply, the words come out more easily, more freely, and with supportive inflection and tone.

Many problems with guiding can be solved by simply breathing deeper. While you are learning the mechanics of guiding the class, finding your natural voice, pinpointing language, and sharpening your skills at touch and support, always come back to your breathing. If you feel tense, anxious, or nervous, deepen your breath. You always have your breath for fuel, comfort, power, and support. Come back to it again and again; with each inhale and exhale, you'll find space to build strength and room to be.

The other thing to keep in mind is that keeping a strong breath-body connection doesn't just support the people in class—it supports us as well. Leading is not just about moving through the sequence. When we breathe deeply, we are able to find the easiest ways to help people—the people in our classes experience simple and challenging moments, and so do we. The focus is just different. They move; we guide. But the breath is at the base of it all.

By grounding yourself in the breath, you can work smarter, and you can avoid a common mishap that ends up draining a lot of Guides: simply pacing back and forth calling out the cues. This idea of yoga teacher burnout when taking on several classes and clients per week happens not from a busy schedule but from an energy drain in approach. If you're burned out from leading, you stop having fun, your energy is zapped, and you are in no position to help. It's okay if it happens—as long as you take it as a sign to change your approach. We know with the easygoing process we can do more with less effort on the mat. The same thing applies to you as the Guide. You can lead more with less effort when you keep deep breathing as a priority. Let your breath do the heavy lifting and carry you to those next amazing places.

LET'S GET FERAL

Let's try a little exercise to get moving as a Guide. This fun practice will help you tap into the breath-body connection and see how to feel ease as you move about the room. You can also do it whenever you feel like you need to loosen up, get back into your body, and fill up with your power source. It's outside the structure of what you would do in a class, but it will help you become more comfortable as you take your position as the leader in the room.

Stand up wherever you are. Step your feet a little wider than hip-width apart. Soften your knees. Relax your shoulders. Get comfortable. Take a few long, deep breaths and let your body move around to get any kinks out. Now start to let your breath move your body. Let your inhales lift you up. Let your exhales move you a little farther. Move from your middle. Let your hips lead the way. Stay connected to your center. The goal here is to feel your breath moving your body. Don't worry about what the movement looks like; start to let your breath move you.

After a few big, deep breaths here, let yourself move around the room guided by your breath. Let the inhales lift and move your body and your exhales soften and move you a little farther. The inhales are your strength, your power, your rise. The exhales are for riding the wave in, moving a little farther, softening into a new space. Let your inhales and exhales be equally powerful. Get creative. Be a creature. Explore around in your body with your breath, and let yourself feel.

Now let's add the voice. Don't worry so much about what you're saying; just let it come out with the feeling of lifting and softening with your inhales and exhales. We're going for raw feeling here; we'll boil it all down to useful instruction after we go wild. Some ideas for phrases: "Big inhale fill up" as you sweep your body upward. "Easy exhale settle" as you glide your body downward. Use equal emphasis on the inhale and exhale to gain a balanced, circular feeling. Go a little wild. You can't do this one wrong. Keep breathing really fully and deeply.

How did that feel? It's pretty great to let yourself get swept away in the power of your breath moving your body. Now let's shift this to another place. Stay with that feeling and deep breathing, and now let your movements cover space without looking so feral. Let yourself carry the awareness of the breath from the exercise and take it into your natural environment where you are walking around. Can you imagine that guiding a class from this place would be useful? Let yourself be easy, calm, relaxed, and soft as you move. Let yourself be lifted and energized by your inhales and moved farther by your exhales.

When we get together with a group of Guides, it's fun to do this together and take up the space moving across the room. It's an exercise designed to get you in your body fueled with your breath. You can even do this with practitioners, but I wouldn't recommend that you use it as part of a normal class.

BREATH-BODY LANGUAGE

When it comes to leading the breath-body connection, it's important to keep the language clear, fresh, and informative—just as I noted in Chapter 7. To figure out effective ways to lead, think of what's happening when we breathe in and what is happening when we breathe out. The inhale lifts, expands, and gets us from a place of not moving to moving. It does the work, the carrying, and the hauling of the body. Using the inhale to move takes the tension away from the body and mind and carries us efficiently where we want to go. The exhale moves us a little farther into a settling moment, a twist, or an opening. The exhale is the moment where we soften and let go. Our minds become calm, allowing our bodies to release tension.

An inhale is like opening the door, and the exhale is like walking through. The deeper and fuller you breathe, the farther you go.

One hint that I like to give is to avoid the words *up* and *down* more than once during the same movement phrase. Using these often makes people feel less expansive, as if they are being forced into two dimensions. Avoiding *up* and *down* will make your movements feel circular, without end points, and expansive. Try it out. Inhale lift. Exhale down. Inhale lift. Exhale down. Try that a few times, and you'll feel yourself shrink. Now try something more circular and see if the feeling and physicality shift. Inhale lift. Exhale soften. Inhale fill up. Exhale settle. Feels different right? The goal is to feel, so keep the language super clear and descriptive and based in feeling.

Now let's look at some phrases that I like to use. We'll do the simple movement of going from warrior 2 to warrior 2 lift and then back to warrior 2.

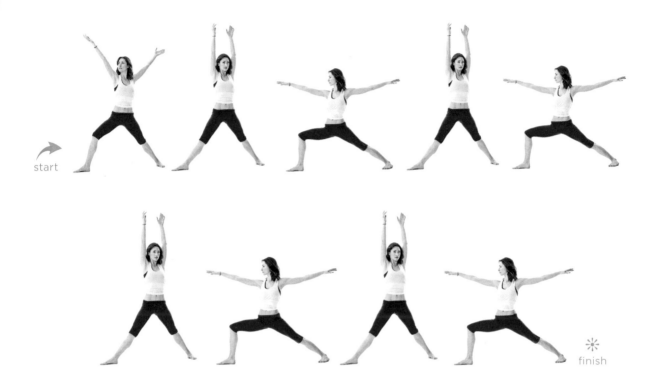

start

finish

1. Inhale lift your hips and arms up. Exhale soften back to warrior 2.

2. Big inhale fill up. Exhale settle back to warrior 2.

3. Big inhale open up lift your hips and arms. Exhale relax to warrior 2.

4. Big inhale fill up the space. Exhale drift back to warrior 2.

5. Take a big inhale and lift your hips and arms way up. Easy exhale and soften back to warrior 2.

Each of these provides very clear frame-by-frame instruction of actions supported by the breath. For example, in the last one, "take a big inhale" is the breath cue. "Lift your hips and arms way up" is the action cue. "Easy exhale" is the breath cue and "soften over your legs" is the action cue. You want to be sure when guiding the breath that you are combining action and breath.

All right! Now it's your turn. Get that journal and write down five ways you can effectively instruct the inhale and exhale. Think of the simplest, most effective instructions using the fewest words. When you boil down your language, you create space for the people in your class to have space in their minds as well. Think of this as an exercise in Hemingway. Be direct, to the point, and ever so descriptive.

Keep in mind that you don't want to cue every inhale and exhale. If you do this, your guiding starts to feel lurching and robotic. You lose the flow of the movements. For example, in a flow through several movements, you'd want to choose to use "inhale lift up" or "inhale open your torso" or "exhale soften over your legs" or "exhale twist to the right" when you are accomplishing bigger movements. Think of the choice of "inhale" and "exhale" as fuel. Sometimes you need fuel, and sometimes you're coasting or exploring. Of course, you are always breathing with the movement, which provides your pacing. When guiding movement, using the word *inhale* comes along with a movement that the inhale lifts you to, like "inhale lift your hips and arms up." The exhale comes along with a movement that takes you to the next place, like "exhale soften back to warrior 2."

As another example of a simple flow where it would be monotonous to repeat inhale and exhale with each movement, here is a language suggestion that works.

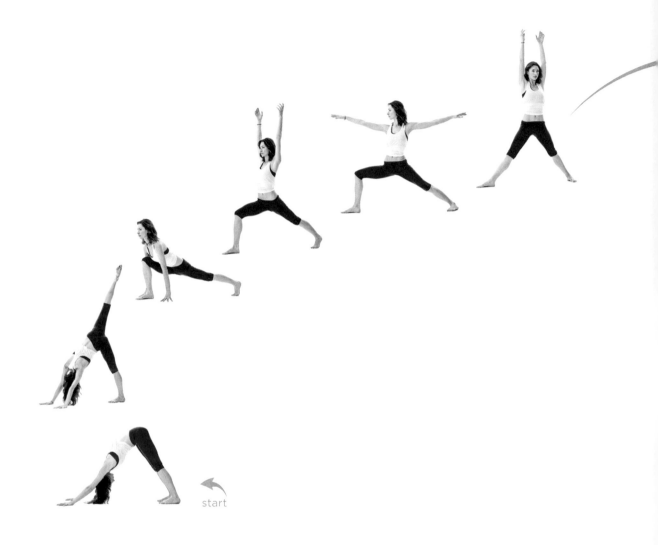

start

Come into down dog. Sway a bit here and settle in for a moment. When you're ready, take a *big inhale and lift* your right leg up and back to down dog split. Open your hips and shoulders if that feels nice. *Exhale and step* your foot on through to low lunge. Press down through your legs and lift up to high lunge. Roll your back heel down and open into warrior 2. Settle here for a moment. Take a *big inhale and lift* your hips and arms up. *Exhale soften back* to warrior 2. Tip back reverse warrior. Tip up and over to your extended side angle,

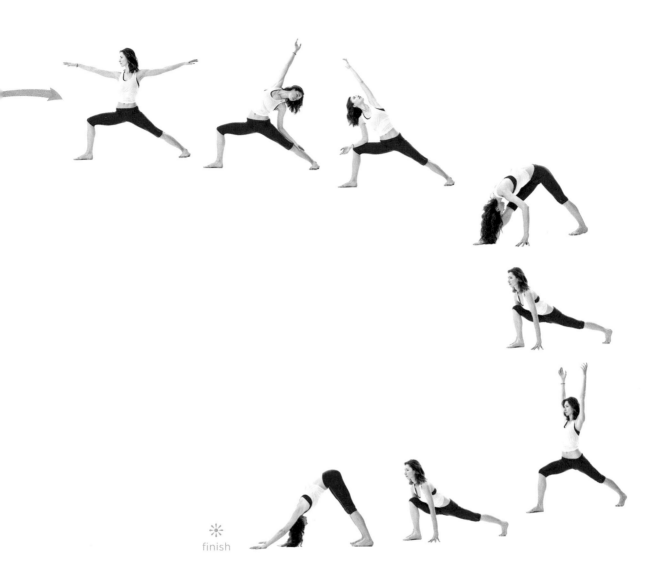

finish

pressing your forearm to your thigh and opening your opposite arm up and overhead. Roll your belly open here. When you're ready, bring your fingertips to the ground on either side of your front foot and sink your hips. Press down through your fingertips and lift your hips up and relax your torso over your front leg. Soften back to low lunge. Press down through your legs, take a *big inhale and lift up* to high lunge. *Exhale soften back* to low lunge and make your way back to down dog.

Using the inhale and movement cue and the exhale and movement cue when you are covering some distance and need the fuel adds stability and also teaches you and the group how to conserve energy and move efficiently with grace and ease. Play around in your own practice, guiding yourself through with putting the inhales and exhales where you think they naturally fit. You'll find those places through exploration and practice.

When you practice your breath-body language, it's useful to guide aloud what you would you say as you do the movements. This will help you see if your language and movements match up with the breath timing. If you are coming up with too much to say that doesn't fit with the breath and the movement, look at what you can edit out of your description. If your descriptions feel choppy or not descriptive enough, go back to the breath and the movement to find what's missing. If you get stuck, go back to a breath cue followed by the movement instruction for each moment and try it on for size from there.

And remember, you need to keep your own breathing in mind, softening and breathing as you instruct. If you just spoke the words without breathing or with a stiff body, arms tight by your side, pacing around the room, the feeling would be rigid and stiff for the people in the class.

THE POWER OF THE GROUP

After just a bit of experimentation here with the breath-body connection and some practice orchestrating, we can feel how much of a difference the breath makes. We are supported, encouraged, and able to connect inward with the use of the breath. This breathing business, although simple, natural, and something we're doing all day long, takes a lifetime to master. The more we place our attention on the breath, the fuller our experience becomes. We come to yoga to feel a connection to our body, our mind, and our purpose in life.

When we come together in groups to practice these elements, it's amazing to see that the clarity of feedback and the experience of breath are universal. Without the breath the group reports feeling anxious, watching the time pass, and feeling controlled by the Guide, unbalanced, wobbly, and uninspired. A Guide shared with the group in a recent training that she felt like the life of her movements was missing without the breath. That's spot on. We can certainly do the movements without using the breath, but we miss the vitality and the spirit when we do so.

With clear, supportive breath-body connection in language, body position, tone, and attitude, people feel carried gently, as if by a wave, during the simple and challenging moments alike. Movement shifts from linear tasks to be accomplished, to a circular journey with no end points. Space is created, and there are endless possibilities for expansion. Take a big, deep breath, come back for more and more, and you'll always be nicely enjoying the flow, not only of the yoga class but also of your soul.

GUIDING FEELING

Now let's move on to feeling. In Chapter 7 we talked about the need to guide action rather than feeling—and that is still true, even in a section called "Guiding Feeling." As a Guide, we don't want to tell people to feel certain things. That closes them in to paying attention to only what we're noting. Our goal is to inspire introspection by slipping in reminders to feel—in general.

Phrases like "if it feels nice," "if it feels good," "settle here for a moment," and "feel around in this position," remind people that they should tune in to their body and adjust themselves in a way that feels good. Grab your journal now and come up with some phrases that feel natural for you. Write down a few "reminder to feel" phrases that roll off your tongue effortlessly.

The effect of our language should be to create space for people to do exactly what they need in that moment. But it's not enough to tell people to feel their way into the movements; we also need to be in feeling mode ourselves. Just as with breathing, it all goes back to that first circle of practice: being.

We have to be connected, feeling, and sensitized. We have to carry ourselves in a way that helps people simply through proximity. We have to inform the people in the class, by our presence alone, that this is a safe place to feel. If we walked around the room guiding feeling but weren't feeling ourselves, something would feel off. The instructions would be experienced more like options. Do this or do that. Do this if you can. If you can't, do that. We want to guide people safely through a structure to choose the path that feels best for them. We acknowledge that choice will be different for each person in the room, and that's wonderful. We are different from day to day, class to class, side to side, so we must tune in to ourselves to understand how to respond accordingly.

Let's bring these ideas into the practice and leading. There are a couple of buckets to organize this giant category of "reminder to feel" into when it comes to the experience of the class. They are "keeping the train moving" and "opportunities to explore." Keeping the train moving means that we're in a movement phrase where it is appropriate to go from one place to another, keeping the flow going. This is appropriate when you put certain movements together. But there are also places where it makes sense to stop and feel around in your body a bit. These are the places to explore. These are places where you stay for a few deep breaths and search for what feels good. Both of these areas offer chances to feel, and effective cuing is required for optimal support.

KEEPING THE TRAIN MOVING

Just like a train continues to move steadily toward its destination, movement phrases can progress along without interruption. I like the train image for the sheer pleasure of enjoying the view of the countryside while you ride along, but the idea of keeping movements flowing works with many metaphors. If you can find one that you like better, go for it. You could talk about a car on an interstate versus in a city. If you've ever been in a cab in New York City, you've probably experienced a fast ride with a lot of sudden stops and starts. Cabbies love to get you to your destination as fast as possible and will cut people off, race through lights, switch lanes suddenly, and then slam on the breaks all within five city blocks. This is the opposite of what we want our class to feel like. Keeping the train moving, or the taxi cruising, is closer to our feeling. The breath lifts, the body follows, and we keep it flowing.

Let's try out a brief movement phrase that keeps the train moving. You may recognize this from Part I—when I took you through the "experience feeling" exercise. We're doing pretty much the same moves here, but this time, I've highlighted the reasons for the cues in bold, dark blue—just to add a little more insight. Take your time to feel as you go through, and really notice the cuing that's happening.

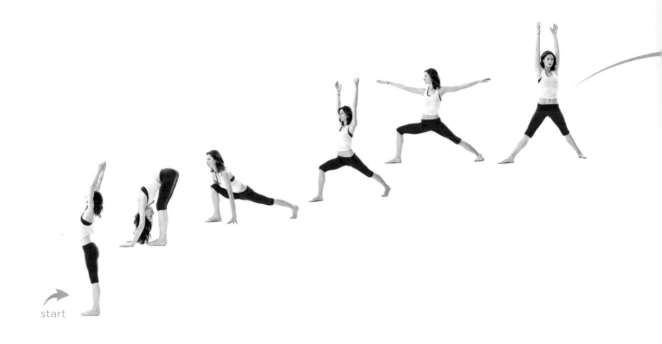

start

Start standing easy, soften your knees a bit here. **Softening before we move**, take a big inhale and lift your arms up. **Lifting up on the inhale, creating space**, exhale and soften over your legs into a forward bend. **Softening and moving into the space**, soften your knees, press your fingertips on the ground, and step your left leg back to a low lunge. Press down through your legs, take a big inhale, and lift up into a high lunge. **Lifting up and creating space**, ground your back heel down and soften into warrior 2. **Moving into the space settling in warrior 2**, take a big inhale and lift your hips and arms up. **Letting the breath lift the body**, exhale and soften back into warrior 2. **Letting the breath soften the body**, take a big inhale and tip back to reverse warrior. **Inhale lifts body moves back**, bring yourself up and over, pressing your right forearm on your thigh and opening your left arm up and overhead rolling your belly open. **Exhale softens up and over, no need to say** exhale **here, it's happening naturally**, bring your fingertips on the ground on either side of your front foot, coming into low lunge. Plant your palms on the ground and step back to plank. **Inhale lifts you up and back to down dog**, take a big inhale and lift your hips up and back to down dog. Take an easy stroll up to the top of your mat one step at a time. Once you make it up relax your torso over your legs. Round up to stand one notch at a time. **Breath happens naturally for these movements so no need to cue. Cuing breath when it's not necessary gives a robotic stuck feeling we want to avoid.** Take a big inhale and lift your arms up. Exhale and soften back over your legs. Repeat the whole phrase on your other side.

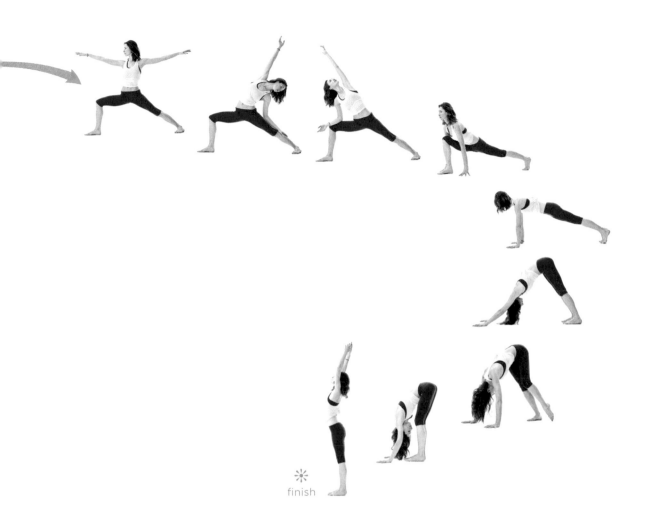

finish

How did that feel? Did you notice how effective the reminder-to-feel cues were? Or perhaps, more accurately, did you notice how there were no specific cues to feel? Yet you still managed to tune in to how you were feeling? When you're keeping the train moving, the cues that inspire feeling aren't overt. They simply come back to the breath, and this opens the space to feel. The breath lifts and the body follows. They're all meant to help people slow down, soften, and breathe deeply. These are the ideas that lead you right to feeling when you're flowing. Telling people to "just feel" or "let it go" or other flowery feeling cues sort of dance around the idea without delivering a direct experience.

OPPORTUNITIES TO EXPLORE

Now let's look at cuing feeling when we reach some opportunities to explore. Remember, these are capsulated experiences where it makes sense to breath in one position for a while. To take a few deep inhales or exhales.

To get us started here, let's take a look at the phrase we worked through above and change it a bit to have some capsulated places to play with.

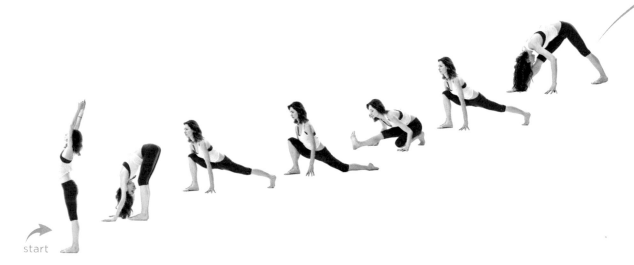

start

Start standing easy, soften your knees a bit here. *Softening before we move*, take a big inhale and lift your arms up. *Lifting up on the inhale, creating space*, exhale and soften over your legs into a forward bend. *Softening and moving into the space*, soften your knees, press your fingertips on the ground, and step your left leg back to a low lunge. Ease your back knee down. If it feels nice to hang your torso low, go for that. If it feels nicer to open up your torso, go for that, breathing really big and fully and deeply. *Gives option on where and how to explore and reminder to breathe deeply.* When you're ready, *allows people to move in their own time within the process*, bring your hips back toward your back heel for your runner's stretch. Relax your torso over your front leg. Sway a bit side to side if that feels nice. *Gives direction on where and how to explore.* When you're ready, *allows space for people's own timing*, crawl yourself back out to your low lunge. Press your fingertips down, lift your hips up, and fold your torso over your front leg. Sway a bit side to side if that feels nice. *Gives direction on where and how to explore*, when you're ready, *allows space for people's own timing*, press down

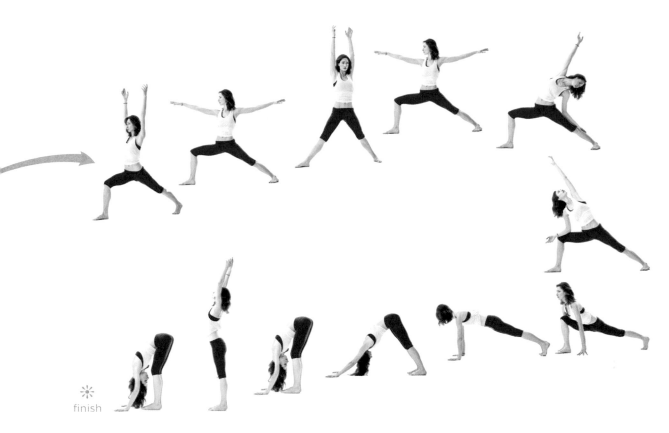

※
finish

through your legs, take a big inhale, and lift up into a high lunge. *Lifting up and creating space*, ground your back heel down and soften into warrior 2. *Moving into the space settling in warrior 2*, take a big inhale and lift your hips and arms up. *Letting the breath lift the body*, exhale and soften back into warrior 2. *Letting the breath soften the body*, take a big inhale and tip back to reverse warrior. *Inhale lifts body moves back*, bring yourself up and over, pressing your right forearm on your thigh and opening your left arm up and overhead rolling your belly open. *Exhale softens up and over, no need to say* exhale *here, it's happening naturally*, bring your fingertips on the ground on either side of your front foot, coming into low lunge. Plant your palms on the ground and step back to plank. Take a big inhale and lift your hips up and back to down dog. *Inhale lifts you up and back to down dog*, take an easy stroll up to the top of your mat one step at a time. Once you make it up, relax your torso over your legs. Round up to stand one notch at a time. *Breath happens naturally for these movements so no need to cue. Cuing breath when it's not necessary gives a robotic stuck feeling we want to avoid.* Take a big inhale and lift your arms up. Exhale and soften back over your legs. Repeat the whole phrase on your other side.

How'd that feel? If you notice the cuing in the section, you'll see that we did things like swaying side to side "if that feels nice." Then we crawled up to low lunge "when you're ready." These types of reminder-to-feel phrases help people remember to tune in to their bodies. To really look at how the position they're in works with them that day. Then they can adjust to what feels better. The opportunities to explore are a more active introspection, and they really provide a concrete step toward sensitization.

FEEL LIKE YOU

It's amazing how different the experience is for tapping into feeling when the cuing feels natural, when it's not flowery or overt, and when it doesn't tell you exactly what to do. Your goal is to inspire people to feel, not to tell them to. It's a different dynamic. It's amazing how empowering guiding this way is. Yoga has a reputation for being intimidating, and one of the reasons that exists is the idea of pose goals. People often feel as if they are doing it right and will get a gold star, which really isn't the point at all. Or they feel they are doing it wrong and become defeated. A yoga teacher might say, "Don't compete" or "Don't judge yourself," but when the feeling cues aren't present for each person to move how it really feels good to move, the elephant in the room is always there. The goal remains the pose until we believe it isn't. The amazing thing that happens when you take the pose goal away is the poses become easy with the process. You become the goal. You'll be able to do more, and the people in your classes will accomplish challenging movements without the struggle. I love when regulars at the studio bring their friends and those friends are blown away by how "great" they are at yoga. Oftentimes our regular isn't even aware that the moves she is doing are hard or supposed to be hard or that she has achieved a perceived challenging pose. She is simply in the process with the practice, and sensitizing to how she feels, which allows her to do more. It makes me smile every time.

GUIDING NATURAL MOVEMENT

Guiding this last piece of the Strala philosophy takes us back into nature—the ebb and flow of movement and the ability to work with your body easily. Obviously, breathing and the reminders to feel in our guiding take us toward moving more naturally. But there are other aspects of guiding that nudge us even closer to the rhythm of nature.

Natural movement, as opposed to technique-based steps needed to achieve a pose, embodies an overall approach of moving easily, with everything you've got, in every direction you can, starting from your center. We don't guide using step-by-step techniques to achieve a position. In fact, we don't aim to "reach a position" at all. Our movements should be circular with no end points.

We avoid the goal of doing something external—turn your thigh, raise your foot, straighten your back—and work to create an internal experience. We focus strictly on the process. We're not trying to get anywhere; we're already here! In this way, Strala brings us directly into the present, rather than trying to be somewhere else.

MOVEMENT PHRASES

You may have noticed throughout the book that I've been using the term *movement phrase* whenever I talk about a group of movements that flow one to the next. I co-opted this term from the dance world to express that we should create movement that is completely fluid, both within each pose and from one to the next. These phrases take you on a journey of movement with the start and end points being attached to a set of movements rather than a single pose. These movement phrases inspire you to move like a tree, swaying with the breeze and moving from the inside out.

This is the biggest part of guiding natural movement. To look at the moves you're bringing in to make sure they create that inspired flow.

How do you do this? Well, look at a move you're doing and then see if the next move flows naturally from it. If you're inhaling and lifting into a high lunge, for example, the exhale will take you a variety of places as options. Maybe you soften right there in a high lunge, softening your knees and elbows a bit to create space for the next lifted high lunge. Or maybe you twist toward your right and open your arms wide. Or perhaps you exhale and bring your thumbs to your heartbeat to prepare for the next inhale. Or maybe you soften to low lunge and head back to down dog. Or you could soften and open to warrior 2. The choices are endless.

Transitions—from one pose to another—are an important focus of natural movement. Unnatural movement starts and stops. It is this pose, and then this pose, and then this pose—all separate things without any attention paid to how you get from one to the next. But with natural movement, it's a flow. Everything is connected, and finding the path of ease during transition from one pose to the next is loads of fun.

MAKING WAVES

When it comes to planning a class, I like to think of it like a glass of water. The glass itself is a solid structure, but the water within moves freely. We're trying to create the glass so people have a safe structure within which they can experience the freedom to flow in a way that's best for them. We do this by giving clear, frame-by-frame guidance, reminding people to feel and to breathe, and promoting natural movement.

To create natural movement, we organize the structure of a class into waves.

The sections of the class feel different, but they flow together with ease. Each class is set up as eight waves. Certain movements are appropriate for the beginning of the class; others make more sense for the middle or the end. There are phrases that are done on one side and repeated on the other side and phrases that are done in the middle. Arranging phrases of rights, lefts, and middles becomes your poetic mission. We've set the stage for the principles, the foundation of the language; next we organize movement phrases together to create the flow. Then we combine the phrases to create a full experience.

Before we dive in and begin to invent, let's review the principles of natural movement because these will guide you as you create your flow.

NATURAL MOVEMENT REVIEW

1. SOFTEN: The softness makes moving possible. Soften before you move so you are working with fluid water, not a solid rock.

2. BREATH-BODY CONNECTION: The inhale lifts and carries your body upward. It gives you strength and fuel. The exhale softens and moves you a little farther, a little easier. It keeps you relaxed and movable.

3. LEAD FROM YOUR MIDDLE. Leading with your breath, soften and move from your middle. Let your hips and belly move first and your arms and legs will follow. This movement will guide your flow.

4. OPPOSITES: Down to go up and left to go right. Apply the concepts of opposites to sustain the lifted energy and access momentum.

5. MOMENTUM: Start with smaller movements and build to larger ones using opposites and everything else.

6. WHOLE BODY: Isolate nothing. You are connected. Move as a whole unit and allow your body to go along for the ride.

7. OPEN DOOR, CLOSE DOOR: One breath to open leads to the next breath to close. Stay in the flow of open and close to avoid running into walls.

8. CONSERVATION OF ENERGY: Use what you need. Rest what you don't. You'll be able to do much more with less effort. Remember, high-performance athletes and animals aren't flexing their muscles to achieve great feats of strength. They gradually increase the scope of what they are able to do by accomplishing everything with the least amount of effort. Flexing muscles to get a workout will only build tense minds and lead to immobilization and underachievement.

9. SENSITIZE: How you move is how you feel. Allow your movement to be a tool to discover what is going on with you.

10. BODY POSITION: Leading with softness to navigate where you are in space is the heart of what you'll be able to do. Can you move easily from where you are? If not, where can you place yourself to create more possibility?

11. PLAY: Having fun is the key to being able to improvise, which is the final secret to mastery. If it's not enjoyable, the task becomes mundane and loses its life. Continually introduce play into what you do and you'll enjoy sustainable lasting energy to accomplish your goals.

CREATING NEW WAVES

When we come together in groups, we spend some time in our own practice, inventing phrases to discover what works and what doesn't work for our classes. Then we get together in smaller groups and invent longer movement phrases so we can check in with our partners about the feeling the phrases give. It's really fantastic to see what's possible when we all play by the same principles. Strala classes aren't meant to be memorized. We start with the principles and invent phrases that are appropriate for the people we are working with.

When it comes to changing up a class sequence, remember that people crave familiarity and the opportunity to work on movements by repetition, class after class, week after week. So replace only one or two waves toward the beginning and middle parts of class, usually when it feels natural after weeks of the same sequence. If someone takes your class every day for six months, he shouldn't notice any drastic changes, but at the end, the class would actually be different from the one he began with. The change should be obvious only to someone who only takes your class every couple of months.

The key is not to trick yourself into believing that changing your class regularly will keep people's interest. You taking an interest in people will keep their interest. The people in your class are different each day, so the class will feel different for each person each day. The familiarity gives people the opportunity to improve and relax in your sequencing. Changing your class and music too often results in people missing the opportunity to work on specific movements and missing the familiarity of the experience they were gaining comfort and space in.

IMPROV EXPERIMENT Ride a Wave

Before you start to plan your classes, let's do an experiment. Taking all you have learned, staying connected to your breath, and paying attention to how you feel, roll out your mat and improvise for 30 minutes or so. See if you can find phrases that feel good to you. See if you can repeat a phrase, add on a bit, and change it a bit while keeping the familiarity. I love the play on theme and variation, and how the element of surprise can come in at just the right time, when we need some relief or a bit of a challenge. Don't think too much about it right now. Just roll out your mat and improvise. We'll refine it all in a bit.

How did your experiment go? Was it fun to freely move around on your mat? What did you discover? Was it difficult to come up with movements to play with, or was it easy? Did you find yourself energized in the flow? Did you come up with any new and interesting phrases you'd like to use for your classes? Did your practice line up with the principles? Take some notes in your journal about anything you experienced—make sure to write down any winning phrases you came up with as you may want to use them later.

STRALA STRUCTURE

Okay, now that we've done some playing, let's get down to the business of structuring a class. Each class begins and ends with three breaths together. The breaths connect us to ourselves and to the group. It's a simple way to sensitize, come together, slow down, and begin.

You'll find a lot of repetition in threes. Three is a magic number in so many ways. Do something once, and it's new. Repeat something again, and it becomes familiar. Try it a third time, and you're at home. Then you can use a single beat of this same movement in the next round to reinforce what you discovered in your threes. By doing this, you breeze through, connecting with yourself and feeling invincible.

Movement phrases can be categorized into two types.

PHRASE TYPE 1: DOUBLE SIDED. These are phrases that happen on one side and then are repeated on the other. Double-sided phrases bring a lot of energy, and they usually begin with a few movements linked together in the first few waves of the class, progressing to longer phrases with more movements toward the middle part of the class, and winding down to a few movements per phrase toward the end. Shorter phrases are simpler and easier to digest physically and emotionally. Longer phrases are exciting and challenging, and they work well to build and maintain energy during the middle part of the class.

PHRASE TYPE 2: EVEN PHRASES. These are movements that happen in the middle. Even phrases are great for calming the energy mentally and physically, even when it's a more advanced class.

When building your own phrases, waves, and classes, look at how you arrange your double-sided and even phrases. Think of yourself as a poet or a composer. A class with all double-sided phrases feels abrasive, while a class with all even phrases feels stuck and uncreative. Alternating evenly from double sided to even would feel predictable, slanting toward boring. It's up to you how to organize your phrases, but I would suggest something along the lines of a few evens, a few doubles, feathered back in with evens and doubles, somewhat predictable to provide familiarity, with an element of surprise thrown in. Try occasionally sandwiching a double sided with an even and see how that feels.

PUTTING YOUR PHRASES TOGETHER TO CREATE ONE BIG WAVE

Another reason for regular practice is continuing to tap into your creativity when it comes to phrases and class design. After putting together a few phrases that make sense, we need to assemble them into the flow of a class. Try improvising on your own to put together phrases that make sense for each wave. Guide yourself through them, speaking out loud with language frame by frame, and see how you can improve your phrase, making it easier to lead and practice. How does it feel? What principles of natural movement did you use to put it together? What is the purpose of your phrase for this part of the class? These are all great questions to ask as you design your classes.

Begin with designing one wave, and keep surfing from there. Make sure the waves build naturally and calm naturally to create a complete experience. Play around and enjoy. Guiding class is like telling an exciting story that only you know the ending to.

I've outlined some classes in Chapter 9 that work for most people in most situations. Versions of these classes are led around the world every day and have wonderful effects, but it's important that your class feels natural to you. Even if you start with these, your class will evolve over time as you become more comfortable. So, try out the phrases in the classes I've outlined, make them your own, and evolve for yourself into what feels like the right dose of familiar and surprise.

BREATHING, FEELING, MOVING, GUIDING

As I'm sure you've figured out by now, the most important lesson in guiding is to get really good at being what you're aiming to guide. The ins and outs of guiding can be refined, but the root always rests in the being. You'll always guide the experience of how you are. If you are breathing and feeling, you guide breath and feeling, which leads to all the exciting benefits of the practice. If you are thinking and posing, you guide an external experience with yoga poses as the goal, which doesn't move you to the freedom and creativity yoga can inspire.

One of the things that I love about guiding Strala is that it isn't about memorizing a script of language or a particular sequence of movements. It's about studying the universal concepts of the breath-body connection, feeling, and natural movement, and how these relate to healing—and then applying this in a way that is natural. The incredible result is that we create such individual classes within a structure of safety, movement, and exploration.

This allows people to move how it feels good to move and accomplish more with less effort, while feeling calm and easy during the whole class. When Guides successfully learn the process, practice, and gain experience, they become comfortable and confident to make a class their own. Supercool, isn't it?

Most systems operate by copying others to retain a familiar experience. But a copy is never as good as the originator, so I've always believed that it's valuable to work with concepts and encourage Guides to access their own uniqueness. That's not to say you play all heavy metal music and do 30 handstands per class. It's a reminder to continue to explore, go deeper into the process, and through practice and improving, your originality will surface naturally. The class feels unique because you are unique and special and talented and amazing.

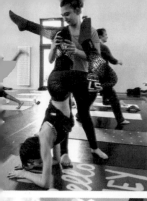

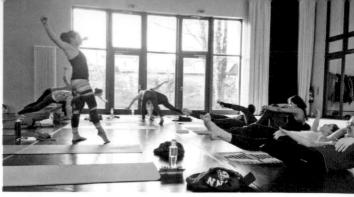
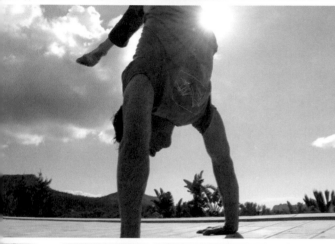
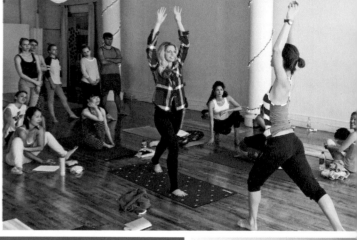
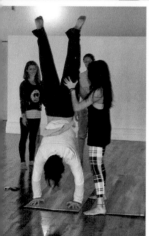

> Yoga is pretty simple.
> It's life that gets complicated.
> So we need to practice in yoga
> what we want in our life.

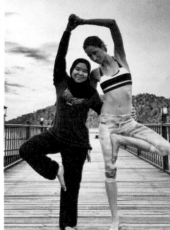
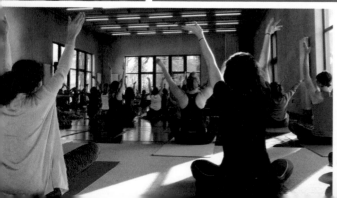
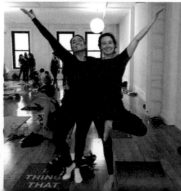

GETTING INTO THE ACTION

SAMPLE STRALA CLASSES

In the classes in this chapter, I have included the language as well as the movement phrases so you can try on and embody the ease with your whole self. I've also suggested places to be in the room for each moment—these are in purple text throughout the chapter. Whether you are in the front demonstrating, on the side demonstrating, or in the group connecting with people, where you are in the room is a part of the clarity of your leading and the effectiveness of your support of the people in your class.

You don't have to work with these classes, but many people like to—just for some comfort. And that's great. Remember, they will change as you gain more experience leading. Even leading the class just as is will still feel unique because you are unique.

Strala isn't about memorizing a sequence; it's about you helping people connect to themselves through a natural process that feels great. Your preparation rests in your regular practice of being. And, of course, I'll keep repeating this over and over until you are sick of it: the most important element to leading is you. Embody what you want to lead. Now, take a big, deep breath, soften, move from your middle, and start leading.

CLASS 1: Strala BASICS

THE PURPOSE

Strala BASICS is designed to build body awareness and familiarity with easygoing, natural movement. It's a great class for anyone new to practicing, and it will build strength and confidence to join any other class. It's also a nice simple class for those with more experience to enjoy.

THE DESCRIPTION

Strala BASICS is a simple flow that releases tension from your body and mind, while resting attention calmly on the breath. You'll build awareness and confidence with the movements to accomplish simple and challenging moments with ease.

FIRST WAVE

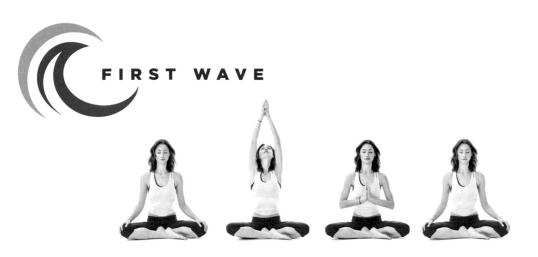

Begin sitting in the front of the room facing the group. Demonstrate along with the group here.

Sit easy, however you can be comfortable. Close your eyes and let your attention rest a bit deeper inward. Take a big inhale and float your arms up and overhead. Press your palms together and bring your thumbs to your heartbeat. Soften here for a moment. All together take a big inhale through your nose. Long exhale out through your mouth. Twice more like that. Big inhale. Long exhale. One more time, big inhale. Long exhale. When you're ready, relax your hands on your thighs.

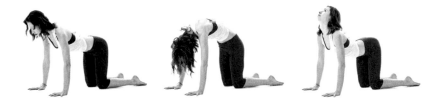

When you guide the group to come into down dog, it's a good time to get up and get involved supporting people. Connecting with people on the lower back is a nice reminder to soften. Remember people can't see or hear you if you are demonstrating a down dog, so it's more useful to get up and get involved here, unless you are in a special circumstance such as leading from a stage to a very large group.

When you're ready, roll out onto all fours, staying easy in your joints and the rest of you. Roll around here a bit however it feels good in your spine, staying easy with your breath. Maybe a bit side to side, or round and round, or forward and back, however feels nice right now.

When you're ready, tuck your toes, take a big inhale, and lift your hips up and back to down dog. Sway a bit here to open up if that feels nice. Pressing into one hand and then the other, shifting your hips from side to side, however feels good to you.

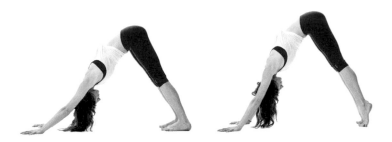

Take a big inhale and lift up onto your tiptoes. Exhale and soften back. Twice more like that: big inhale and lift up. Soften back and relax. One more time, big inhale and lift. Exhale, soften, and relax.

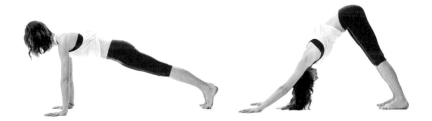

When guiding side plank, it's nice to put yourself to the side where people can see you when they open up. For a side plank on the right hand, standing on the left side of the room as you take the big, deep inhale is a nice reminder. Making your way to the right side of the room (while you are guiding the center plank) for the second side is great also. Remember to move easily in your body as you navigate in the room. Let your voice, body, and breath-body connection support you.

Tuck your chin and round out into your plank, the top of your push-up. Hang here for a moment. Sway a bit side to side or forward and back if that feels nice. When you're ready, lift your hips up and back to down dog.

Lower to belly and back arch works either demonstrating it at the front of the room or demonstrating it with your upper body clearly in the middle of the group and doing the movements as well. If you are demonstrating in the middle of the room, you have more access to connect with people in child's pose and forward bend for a moment of support.

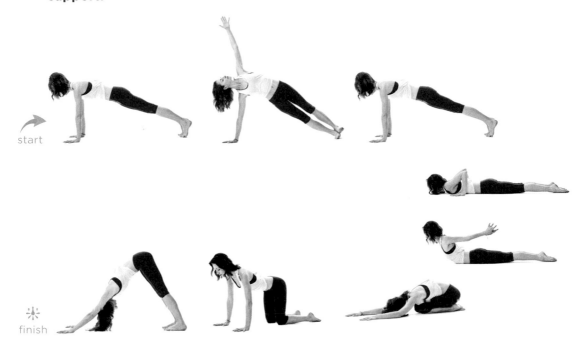

start

finish

Tuck your chin and round out into plank. Lift your hips up a bit, shift your weight onto your right arm and the outside edge of your right foot, and open up to a side plank facing your left side. When you're ready, come back to your middle and open up to your other side. When you're ready, roll back to your plank. Soften your elbows and lower to your belly. Interlace your hands behind you and lift up. Sway a bit here if that feels nice. When you're ready, soften back down. Press your palms on the ground next to your chest and shift your hips back to your heels. Rest here for a moment. When you're ready, come onto all fours, spread your fingers wide, tuck your toes, and take a big inhale to lift up and back to down dog.

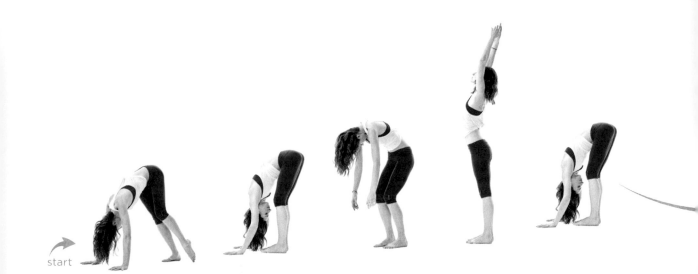

start

You have an opportunity for touch in the standing forward bend. Rolling up to stand is nice to show with your own voice and body facing the group, whether in front of the whole group or in front of a row, depending on where you are. It's nice to show the back arch in your body while you are standing so you're up and mobile and people can see and hear you. From here, you have an easy opportunity to gracefully connect with someone through touch for child's pose and down dog.

Gently walk your feet up to your hands one step at a time. Hands can move too if that feels nice. Once you make it up, soften your torso over your legs. Let your head and neck go. When you're ready, round up to stand one notch at a time.

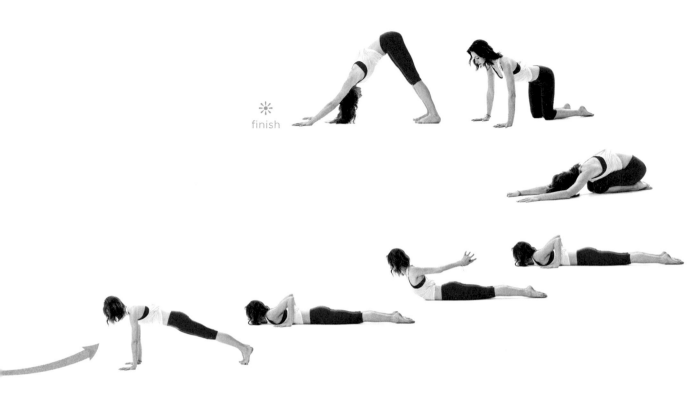

*
finish

Once you make it up, take a big inhale and float your arms out and up. Exhale and soften back over your legs. Twice more like that, round up one notch at a time. Once you're up, take a big inhale and lift your arms out and up. Exhale and relax over your legs. One more time, rounding one notch at a time, big inhale reach your arms out and up. Soften back over your legs.

    Soften your knees, plant your palms on the ground, and step back to plank. Soften your elbows and lower to your belly. Interlace your hands behind you and open your chest up. Sway a bit here if that feels nice. When you're ready, relax back down. Press your palms on the ground, and shift your hips back toward your heels. Rest here for a moment. When you're ready, come back to all fours, spread your fingers nice and wide, tuck your toes, take a big inhale, and lift your hips up and back to down dog.

SECOND WAVE

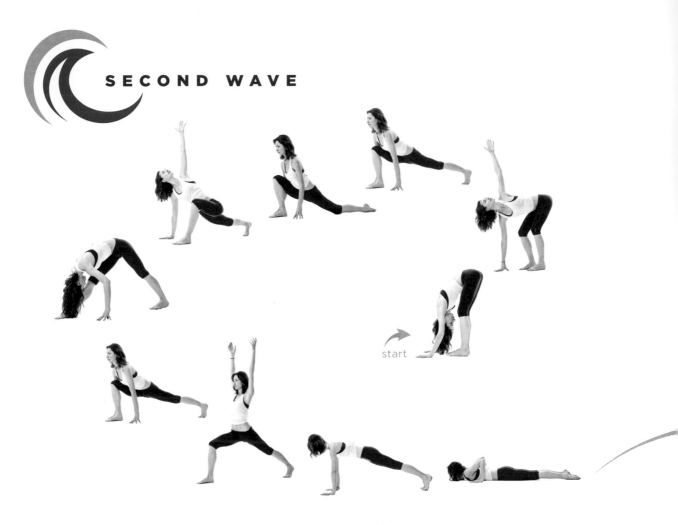

start

This is another place where you could either demonstrate facing and mirroring or be in the room connecting through touch and support.

Walk your feet up to the top of the mat one easy step at a time. No hurry. Once you make it up, soften your torso over your legs. Let your head and neck go. Soften your knees, press your right fingertips on the ground, take a big inhale, and open your body toward your left. When you're ready, soften back to your middle. Press your left fingertips on the ground, take a big inhale and open toward your right. When you're ready, soften back to your middle.

Soften your knees, press your fingertips on the ground, and step your left leg back to your low lunge. Sink your hips low and sway a bit if that feels nice. When you're ready, soften your back knee to the ground and settle here for a moment, breathing really big and fully and deeply. Lean to your right, press your right fingertips on the ground, take a big inhale, and open your body toward your left.

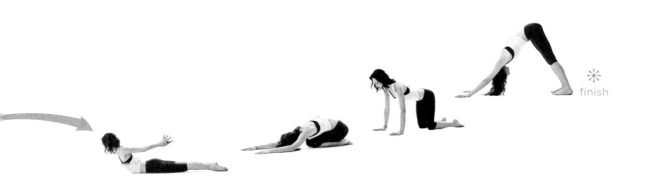

finish

Exhale and soften toward your middle. Press your left fingertips on the ground, take a big inhale, and open to your right. Exhale and soften back to your middle.

Press your fingertips into the ground, take a big inhale, and lift your hips up and relax your torso over your legs. Sway a bit here if that feels nice. Let your head and neck go. When you're ready, sink your hips back to your low lunge. Press down through your legs and lift up to your high lunge. Exhale back down, plant your palms on the ground and step back to plank. Soften your elbows and lower to your belly. Interlace your hands behind you and open up the front of your body. Sway a bit here if that feels nice. When you're ready, soften back down. Plant your palms on the ground and shift your hips back to your child's pose. Settle here for a moment. When you're ready, come onto all fours, spread your fingers wide, tuck your toes, and take a big inhale to lift your hips up and back to down dog.

Repeat the phrase on the other side.

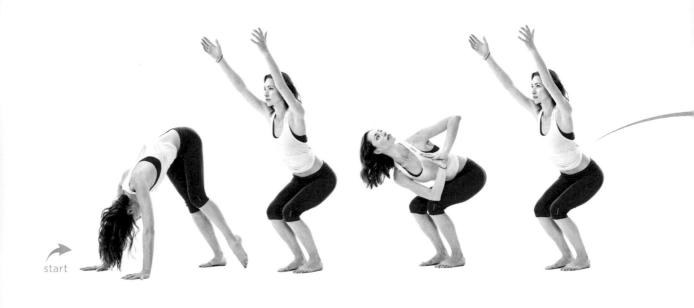

start

Demonstrating chair and this series is a good idea facing and mirroring at the front of the room.

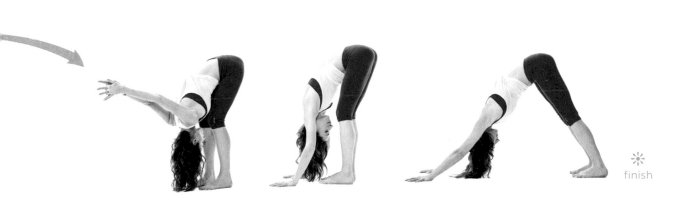

finish

Walk your feet up to the top of your mat, one step at a time. Once you make it up, fold over your legs. Let your head and neck relax. Soften your knees a bit if that feels nice. Sink your hips, take a big inhale, and lift up into your chair pose. Press your palms together, exhale and twist toward your left, pressing your right elbow outside your knee. Take a big inhale and lift up to your chair and twist toward your other side. Take a big inhale back into your chair, exhale and fold up and over your legs, catching your hands behind your back and relax over your legs. Sway a bit here if that feels nice. When you're ready, release your hands, plant your palms, soften your knees, and make your way back to down dog.

THIRD WAVE

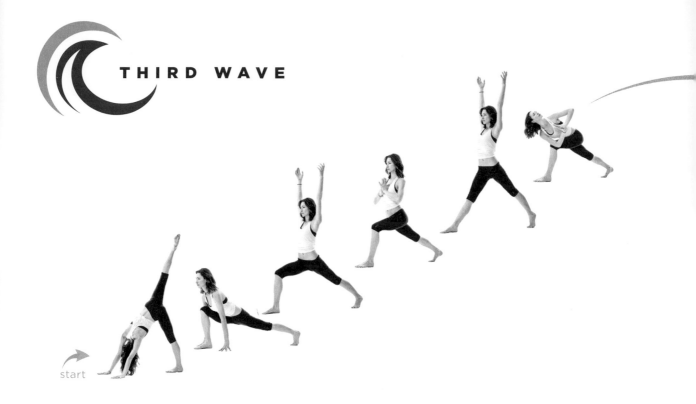

start

Remember people can't see or hear you when you're in down dog, so down dog split to low lunge is a nice movement to guide with your voice and body connection. Head to the front of the room to demonstrate the rest of this phrase after you make it to low lunge. When moving through a longer standing phrase like this, it's useful to demonstrate at the front, facing and mirroring the group to give the visual cue along with your voice and breathing.

Soften in your down dog. Sway a bit here to keep things easy and gentle in your body. Take a big inhale and lift your right leg up and back to down dog split. Open your hips and shoulders if that feels nice. Step your foot between your hands to low lunge. Press down through your legs and lift up to your high lunge. Press your palms together and bring your thumbs to your heartbeat. Take a big inhale and lift, exhale and twist toward your left, bringing your right elbow outside your left thigh. Open up your arms and bring your right fingertips to the ground for support. Take a big inhale, and open up toward your left. When you're ready, bring both fingertips to the ground on either side of your front foot, lift your hips, and relax your torso over your front leg. Sway a bit here if that feels nice. Spin your back heel to the ground and open up

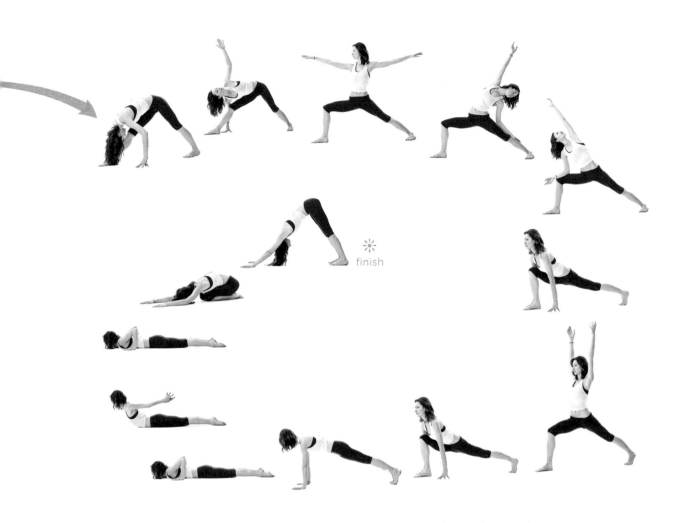

finish

your body to your left side for your triangle. Soften through your knees, press down through your legs, and lift everything up. Lifting your hips and arms up overhead, soften into your warrior 2. Tip back reverse, tip up and over to your extended side angle, pressing your forearm to your thigh. Roll your body open. Bring your fingertips to the ground on either side of your front foot, coming into your low lunge. Press down through your legs, take a big inhale, and lift up to your high lunge. Exhale back to your low lunge, plant your palms, and come into your plank. Soften your elbows and lower to your belly. Interlace your hands behind your back and open up the front of you. Sway a bit here if that feels nice. When you're ready, soften back to your belly. Press your hands on the ground and shift your hips back to your heels. Soften here for a moment. When you're ready, come back onto all fours, spread your fingers wide, tuck your toes, take a big inhale, and lift your hips up and back to down dog.

Repeat the phrase on the other side.

FOURTH WAVE

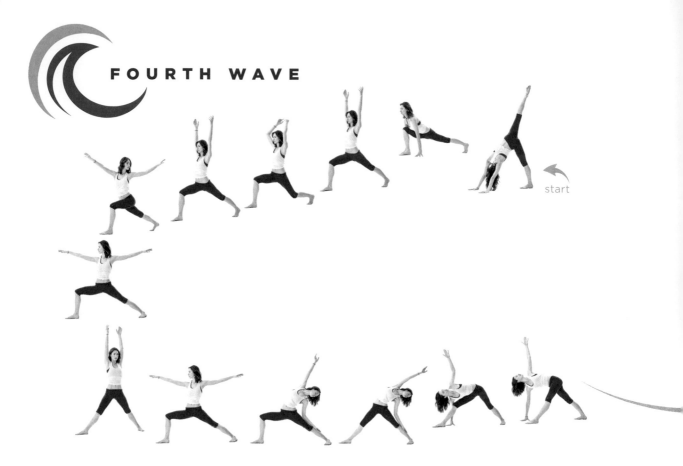

start

Again this is another nice place to be in the front of the room facing and mirroring the group. A hand on the lower back from the side of the person is a nice moment to help someone release tension. When you come back around to guide warrior 3, it's nice to return to the front to face and guide, mirroring again so people can see you. When it's time for down dog, that's your cue to get involved in the group and find someone to connect with through touch if the opportunity presents itself.

Take a big inhale and lift your right leg up and back to down dog split. Open your hips and shoulders if that feels nice. Step your foot on through to low lunge. Press down through your legs and lift up to high lunge. Exhale and soften right here. Inhale and lift up to high lunge. Exhale and twist to your right, let your arms open wide. Big inhale lift up to high lunge. Twice more just like that.

Big inhale and lift up and open to warrior 2. Spin your back heel down and soften your arms out to your sides. Settle here for a moment. Take a big inhale and lift everything up; lift your hips and arms. Exhale soften back to warrior 2. Tip back reverse warrior and lengthen your front leg. Tip up and over to your triangle, soften

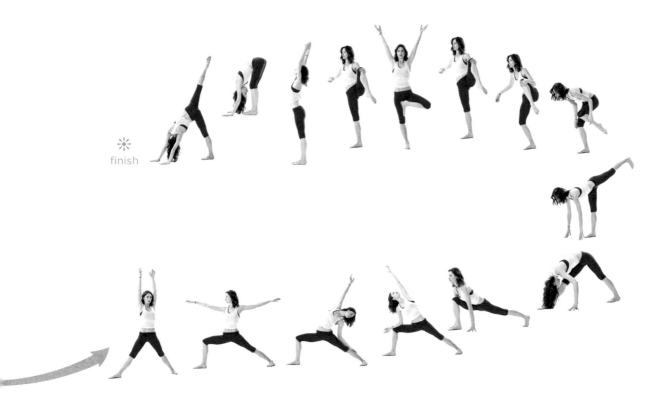

※
finish

your knees and bring your right fingertips to the ground. Take a big inhale and open up toward your left. Soften and bring your left fingertips to the ground, take a big inhale and open up to your right for your twisted triangle. Soften and bring your right fingertips to the ground and open back up to your open triangle. Soften your knees, press down through your legs, take a big inhale, and lift up, lifting your hips and arms up. Exhale and soften to warrior 2. Tip back reverse. Tip up and over to your extended side angle, pressing your right forearm on your thigh and opening your left arm up and over. Roll your body open. Bring your fingertips to the ground on either side of your front foot and sink your hips to your low lunge. Sway a bit here if that feels nice. Lift your hips up, soften your knees, and crawl yourself out into warrior 3. Soften your knees and round up to stand hugging your right shin into your chest for a squeeze. Roll your hips around here if that feels nice. Press your foot into your thigh or onto your ankle for your tree, however is most comfortable. Open your arms up and hang here for a few moments. Sway a bit if that feels nice staying soft and steady. When you're ready, hug your shin back into your chest, take a big inhale, and give it a squeeze. Exhale and soften coming into standing. Soften your knees, take a big inhale, and lift everything up. Exhale and soften into your forward bend. Soften your knees, plant your palms on the ground and make your way back to down dog.

Repeat the phrase on the other side.

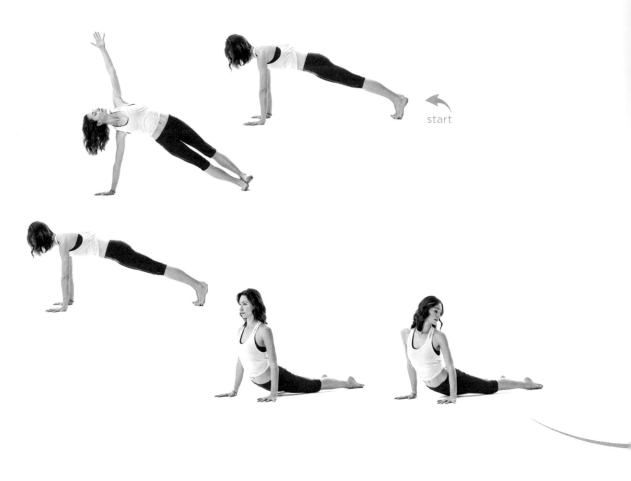

start

For the side planks, putting yourself on the side of the room where people can see you is a great place to be. Guiding through up dog and child's pose from the middle of the room leaves you the opportunity to connect with someone in child's pose and down dog. Going to the front to demo this can work also, but you'll miss the opportunity for touch and support. You can pick it up again with the down dog.

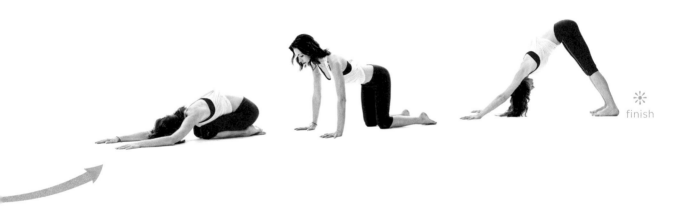

finish

Tuck your chin and round out into plank. Sway a bit here if that feels nice. Shift your weight onto your right side, take a big inhale, and open your body to your left. When you're ready, come back to plank and open to your other side. When you're ready, come back into plank. Soften your knees to the ground and sink your hips into up dog. Sway a bit here if that feels nice. When you're ready, shift your hips to your heels and relax in child's pose. When you're ready, come onto all fours, spread your fingers wide, tuck your toes, take a big inhale, and lift up and back to down dog. Soften here.

FIFTH WAVE

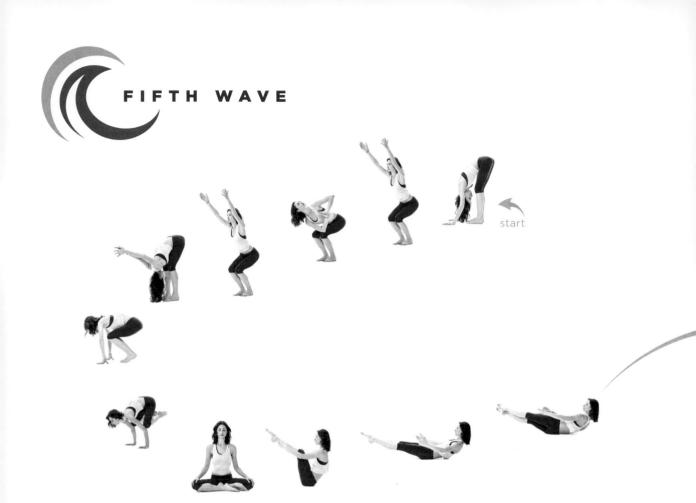

start

Here we have another great phrase for being in front of the group and mirroring. The boat movements are great to mirror for encouragement. When you're doing them along with everyone, it sets a nice vibe of togetherness.

When you're ready, walk on up to the top of your mat. Hands can walk too. Fold over your legs. Soften your knees. Sway a bit here if that feels nice. When you're ready, sink your hips, take a big inhale, and lift up into chair. Press your palms together and twist to your left, bringing your right elbow outside your left thigh. Take a big inhale and lift back up. Easy exhale and twist toward your right. Big inhale and lift up. Exhale and relax up and over your legs. Interlace your hands behind your back and relax over your legs. Sway a bit here if that feels nice. When you're ready, release your hands, press your palms on the ground, put some weight into your arms, and come into a squat. Roll around a bit here to open up how it feels nice. If you'd like to play with your crow, rock back, bringing your hands behind you on

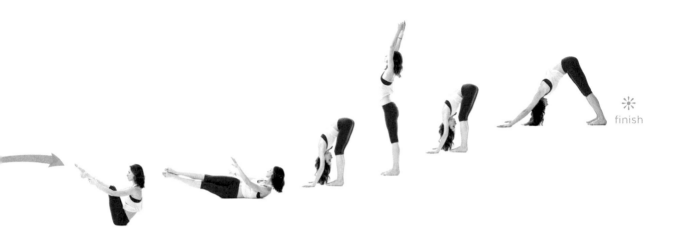

finish

the ground. Take a big inhale and rock forward, planting your palms on the ground. Lean forward and look forward. Exhale, rock back, and relax. Go for that a few times and explore around. When you're ready, bring your hands behind you and come to sit down easily. Lift your legs up into your boat. If this hurts at all, you can always bring your hands behind you on the ground for support. Lower halfway down and all the way back up. Ease on down, and right back up. A few more like that, all the way down, and right back up, soft in your head and neck and shoulders (as we lower down), and right back up. All the way down, and right back up.

Roll down on your right side, and all the way back up. Now over to the left, and right back up. A few more like that, all the way down, and right back up. And all the way down, and right back up. Couple more times, over to the right side, and right back up. Over to the left side, and right back up. Over to the left side, and right back up. Last round, over to your right side, and right back up. Over to your left side, and right back up.

When you're ready, soften your hips and crawl around to a standing forward bend. Soften over your legs. Sway a bit here if that feels nice. When you're ready, round up to stand one notch at a time. When you make it up, take a big inhale and float your arms up. Easy exhale and soften over your legs. Soften your knees, plant your palms on the ground and make your way back to down dog.

SIXTH WAVE

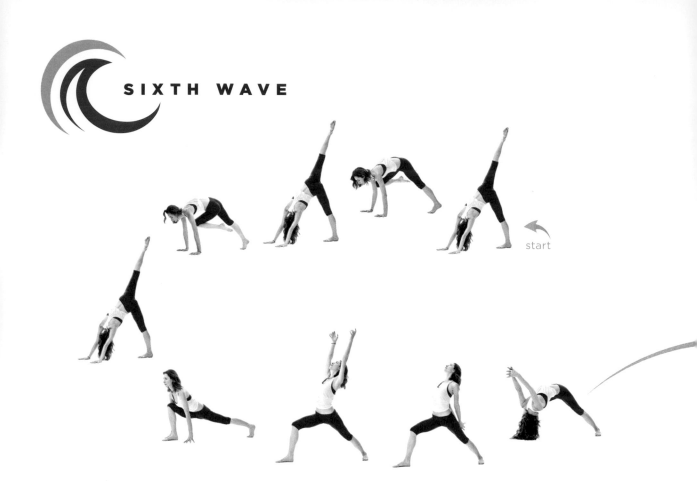

start

The knee hovers and crosses are nice to guide with your voice and breath-body connection as you move around the room. When you meet up in low lunge, it's nice to face, mirror, and demo from there. When you make it to forearm plank, it might be a good opportunity to help people if they are naturally rocking up, or an opportunity to connect with people in child's pose and down dog. You'll find the moments when there is continuous movement and lots of standing phrases make sense to face, mirror, and demo. The moments when there is exploration, like forearm stand, child's pose, pigeon, forward bends, and down dog, are great opportunities to connect and employ your skills of touch and support.

Take a big inhale and lift your right leg up and back to down dog split. Open your hips and shoulders if that feels nice. Arc your knee high and around to your right upper arm. Look forward. Lean forward. When you're ready, lift the leg up and back to down dog split. Arc your knee down and across to your left upper

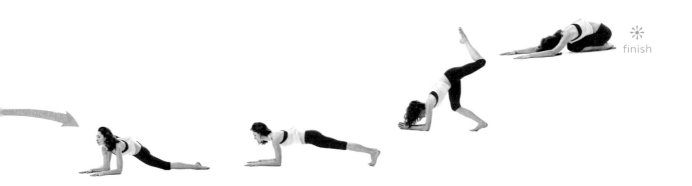

✳ finish

arm. Look forward. Lean forward. When you're ready, lift your leg up and back to down dog split. Step your foot on through to low lunge. Spin your back heel down, press down through your legs and lift up to warrior 1. Soften here. Roll around in your hips and belly to find a good place. Settle here for a few deep breaths. When you're ready, relax your arms down and interlace your hands behind you. Take a big inhale and open up. Exhale and soften, bringing your torso inside your front leg. Press down through your legs, take a big inhale, and lift up. Exhale and soften inside your front leg. When you're ready, relax your hands down to the ground and move your front foot out to the edge of your mat. Soften your back knee down and take some time to get into your hips. Either stay upright or soften your elbows, coming down a bit lower. Move easily so you can find a great place. Sway a bit here if that feels nice. When you're ready, come onto your forearms. Lean toward your left so much that your right leg slides around you to come into a forearm plank. Up to you, either breathe here or walk your feet up toward your face a bit. Take a big inhale and lift a leg, lifting your hips and belly. Exhale soften your leg back down. Roll through that a few times on each side. When you're ready, rest in child's pose for a few deep breaths.

Repeat the phrase on the other side.

GETTING INTO THE ACTION ⬡ 191

SEVENTH WAVE

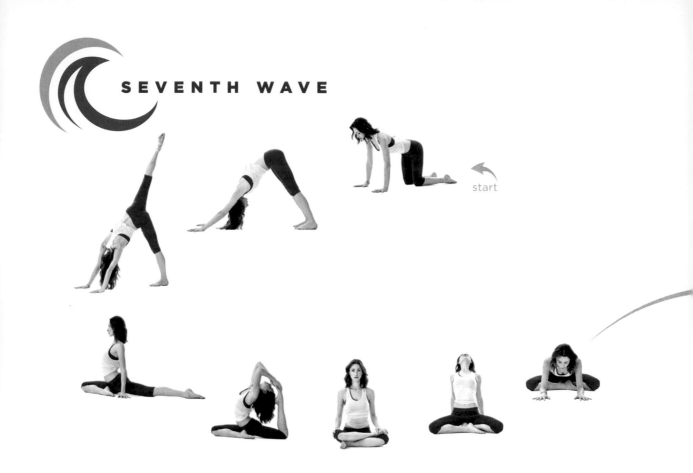

start

Here is a big chance to connect with a few people in pigeon. You have several breaths to spend with each person and might make it to two or three people with the time here. The seated forward bends are nice to demo and mirror how to get into them. If you are spending more than a few breaths in a forward bend, it's nice to get up and connect with touch. If you are doing something here like a gentle twist one way and the other, it's nice to demo and mirror to show the movements and breath.

When you're ready, come onto all fours, spread your fingers wide, tuck your toes, and lift your hips up and back to down dog. Soften here for a moment. Take a big inhale and lift your right leg up to down dog split. Open your hips and shoulders if that feels nice. Soften your shin on through for your pigeon. Take a moment to get comfortable here. Roll around a bit to find a place where you feel a good opening and can breathe fully. If you feel good here, hang here. If you'd like to take a big inhale and open up, go for that. Either hang here or guide yourself on forward. Crawl around to one side and the other, finding a place where you can settle for a while. Take several long, deep breaths here. When you're ready, bring your-

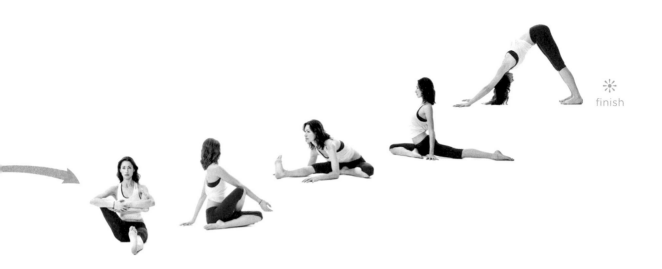

finish

self back up. Lean toward your front hip and bring your back leg around, stacking your ankles and knees if that feels nice or bringing your left leg in front of your right for an easy cross-legged seat. Bring your hands behind you on the ground and lean back and open. Either stay here if this feels nice or explore your way on forward, crawling around to one side and the other, finding a nice place to settle for a bit. Hang here for a few long, deep breaths. When you're ready, bring yourself back up. Grab hold of your top shin, hugging it toward you. Sway a bit side to side if that feels nice. Lengthen your bottom leg out in front of you. Take a big inhale and give the shin a squeeze; exhale and cross it over your extended leg. Take a big inhale and lift your right arm up; exhale and cross it over your left leg. Bring your left fingertips behind you on the ground. Take a big inhale and lift up tall, exhale, and twist around a little farther. Hang here for a few deep breaths. When you're ready, unwind toward the other side. Bring your foot on the ground inside of your extended leg. Relax your hands on the ground beside you. Take a big inhale and open up; exhale and soften over your extended leg. Sway a bit here if that feels nice. When you're ready, bring yourself back up. Hug your shin back in, slide your bottom leg back, and wind your way back to your pigeon. Plant your palms on the ground and make your way back to down dog however feels nice for you. Take your time unwinding this side. Roll through some cat cows, or stretch one leg up and back, or shift your weight from one side to the other in down dog, or do something else that feels good for you. We'll meet in down dog in a bit.

Repeat the phrase on the other side.

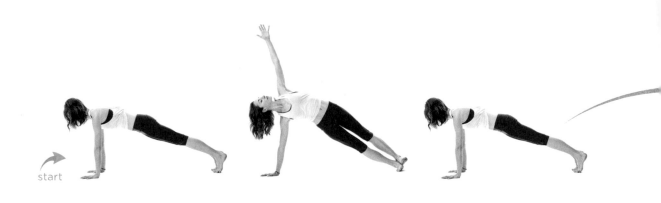

start

For your side planks, it's nice to be on the side where people are facing so they can see you. You have an opportunity for touch in child's pose and down dog.

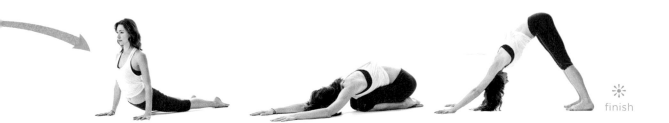

finish

Tuck your chin in toward your chest and round to plank. Shift your weight onto your right side, take a big inhale, and open to your left. When you're ready, come back to the middle and open to your other side. When you're ready, come back to your plank, soften your knees to the ground, and sink your hips to your up dog. Sway a bit here if that feels nice. Keeping your knees on the ground, bring your hips to your heels and relax in child's pose for a few deep breaths. When you're ready, come back to all fours, spread your fingers wide, tuck your toes, and take a big inhale and lift up into down dog.

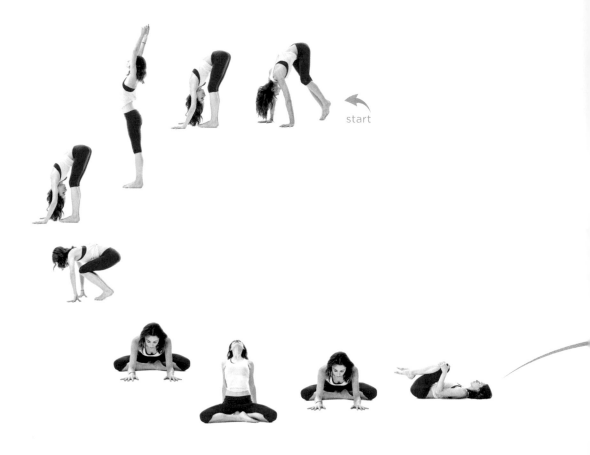

start

Another opportunity comes up with forward bend. It's nice to demo the rolling up and down and coming into a squat. For knee safety reasons, make sure to show bringing the weight into your arms as you come into the squat. Remember, people will do what you do more than what you say. Coming into a squat without the support of the hands is precarious on your knees, and safety is our first rule. Do no harm. It's nice to show choices for forward bends and then get up and connect with someone through touch. You can guide the winding down with your voice and breath-body connection.

When you're ready, walk on up to the top of your mat, one step at a time. Hands can walk too. Once you make it up, fold up and over your legs. Soften your knees and sway a bit if that feels nice. Round up to stand one notch at a time. Once you make it up, take a big inhale and float your arms out and up. Exhale and soften up and over your legs.

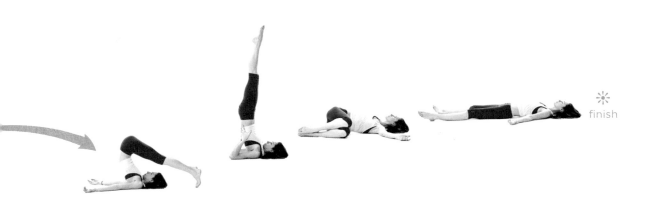

finish

When you're ready, release your hands, press your palms on the ground, put some weight into your arms, and come into a squat. Roll around a bit here to open up how it feels nice. When you're ready, bring your hands behind you and come to sit down easily. Do any forward bend that feels nice to you, feet together, legs apart, or forward. Take a big inhale and lean back and open up. Either stay here if this feels nice or guide yourself forward, exploring around to one side and then the other, finding a nice place to breathe for a few moments. When you're ready, round on down to your back, carrying your knees along with you. Hug your knees into your chest and either rock side to side to open up or round up and over for your plow. If plow doesn't feel nice on your back and neck, round gently down. If you'd like to evolve your plow into your shoulder stand, bring your palms to support your back and lift your legs up. Wherever you are, breathe really fully and deeply. Feel free to stay there as long as feels nice. When you are ready, ease on back down. Anything else you'd like to roll through before we rest. Maybe a gentle twist side to side. Take your time. When you're ready, stretch out a bit. If there is any tension lingering, take a big inhale in through your nose and a long exhale out through your mouth. Twice more just like that. When you're ready, rest here.

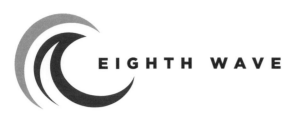

EIGHTH WAVE

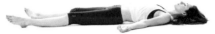

Here you have an opportunity to connect with several people through touch. There's nothing to guide with words here. Moving around the room supporting people with touch is great.

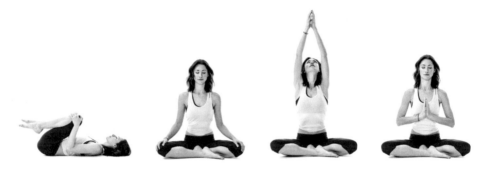

It's great to be in the front of the room sitting easily as you guide people to come out of the relaxation and meeting them in easy seated for meditation.

Start to invite some more air back into your body. Roll around your wrists and ankles if that feels nice. Stretch out your arms overhead if that feels nice. When you're ready, hug your knees into your chest, and make your way up to sit in the easiest way.

Close your eyes and let your attention drift inward. Take a big inhale and float your arms up and overhead. Press your palms together and bring your thumbs to your heartbeat. Soften here for a moment. Take a big inhale through your nose. Exhale out through your mouth. Twice more like that, big inhale. Long exhale. One more time, big inhale, long exhale. Soften here for a moment.

Namaste and thank you for coming!

CLASS 2: Strala GENTLE

THE PURPOSE

Strala GENTLE is designed to provide a simple and expansive framework for the experience of ease. The aim is to softly wake up and sensitize the body and mind to and build awareness through easygoing movement and meditation. It's a great class for anyone interested in feeling the whole body and mind without the component of physical challenge.

THE DESCRIPTION

Strala GENTLE is an easygoing flow that softly wakes up and sensitizes the whole body and mind while building awareness through meditative movement. You'll build focus and clarity through the simplicity of ease.

FIRST WAVE

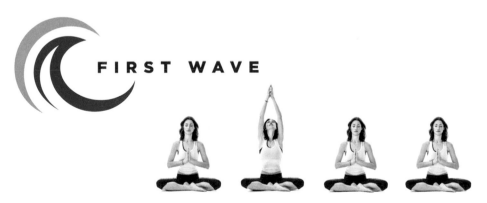

Begin sitting in the front of the room facing the group. Demonstrate along with the group here.

Sit easy, however you can be comfortable. Close your eyes and let your attention rest a bit deeper inward. Take a big inhale and float your arms up and overhead. Press your palms together and bring your thumbs to your heartbeat. Soften here for a moment. All together take a big inhale through your nose. Long exhale out through your mouth. Twice more like that. Big inhale. Long exhale. One more time, big inhale. Long exhale. When you're ready, relax your hands on your thighs.

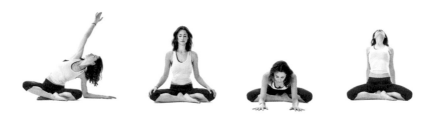

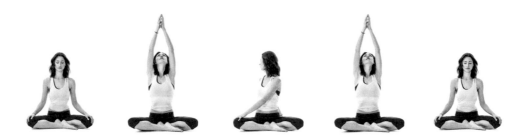

This is great to demonstrate mirroring and facing the group.

Tip over toward your right side, bringing your left forearm to the ground. Open your right arm up and overhead. Sway a bit here if that feels nice. When you're ready, bring yourself back up to the middle. Same thing other side, tipping over, keeping both sides of your waist nice and long. When you're ready, bring yourself back up through center. Crawl yourself forward a couple steps or a few more if that feels nice. Let your head go. Let your neck go. Sway a bit here if you want. When you're ready, bring yourself back up through center. Bring your fingertips behind you on the ground and lift up. Lift your hips up also if that feels nice. When you're ready, bring yourself back to center. Rest your palms on your thighs, close your eyes, and let your attention drift back inward.

Take a big inhale and float your arms out and up. Bring your left hand on your right knee and right fingertips behind you on the ground. Take a big inhale and lift up. Exhale and twist around a bit. Stay here for a few long, deep breaths. When you're ready, bring your back arm up and around, grabbing hold of opposite knees. Relax your head, neck, and torso. Sway a bit here if that feels nice. When you're ready, bring yourself back upright. Take a big inhale and float your arms out and up. Repeat the twists on the right and left sides once more.

When you're ready, bring yourself back to center. Rest your hands on your thighs and close your eyes. Let your attention drift inward. When you're ready, open your eyes.

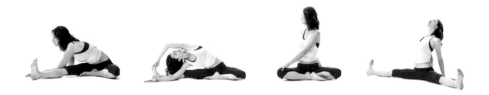

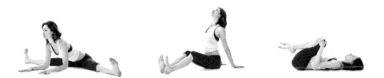

This is nice to demonstrate mirroring and facing. If you are clear in your language, it's also a great place to get up and use touch and support for the forward bends.

Extend your right leg out to your side, keeping your left leg tucked in. Soften your right knee and lean over toward your right, bringing your right hand on the ground next to your right leg. Open your left arm up and over toward your right leg. If you happen to grab hold of your right foot with your left hand, use the grip to roll around a bit. Hang here for a few long, deep breaths. When you're ready, roll on up, unwinding with a twist. Bring your right hand to your left knee and your left fingertips behind you for an easy twist. When you're ready, come back to center and gently switch the legs. Repeat the side stretch on the opposite side.

When you're ready, roll on up, unwinding with a twist. Bring your left hand to your right knee and your left fingertips behind you for an easy twist. When you're ready, come back to center. Open both legs out to your sides a bit. Soften your knees. Bring your fingertips behind you on the ground, take a big inhale, and open up a bit. Stay here if this feels nice or crawl yourself forward a bit. Explore around one side and the other, finding a nice place to rest for a few deep breaths. When you're ready, bring yourself back up. Bring both legs out in front of you, keeping your knees soft. Bring your fingertips behind you on the ground and open up a bit. Either stay here or crawl yourself gently forward. Sway a bit here if that feels nice. When you're ready, round on down to rest on your back, bringing your knees along with you for the ride to go easier on your back. Hug your knees into your chest and rock a bit side to side.

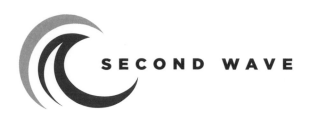

SECOND WAVE

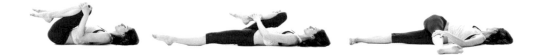

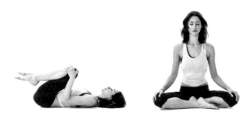

This is a good time to get up and connect with the people in the class. You can support with the twists side to side as you make your way through the room. There is no need to be up front when people are on their backs because they won't be able to see or hear you. Remember it's always best to be where people can see and hear you so you can be useful for demonstration or provide contact with support.

Keep hold of your right shin and let your left leg drift down toward the ground. Roll around the right leg a bit to open up the hip. Either stay here if this is enough of an opening or take an easy twist, letting your right leg drift over toward your left side. Arms can open out to your side. Either gaze upward or over toward your right side if that feels nice. Hang here for a few long, deep breaths. When you're ready, bring your right leg back into your chest and switch legs.

When you're ready, bring your knees back to your chest, hug both knees in, and rock a bit side to side. Take your time and find an easy way to come back to sitting. Close your eyes, rest your hands on your thighs, and draw your attention inward. Soften here for a few moments. When you're ready, gently open your eyes.

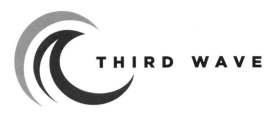

THIRD WAVE

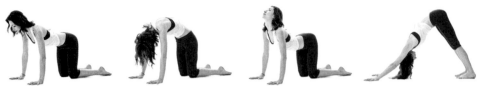

Demonstrate facing and mirroring; sit to one side to come around onto all fours instead of coming through the middle over your knees. It's a big deal for knee safety not to roll over the knees in this position. What may be easy for you might blow out someone else's knee with a different build or old sports injury. Move gently as you demonstrate.

Staying easy, make your way gently to all fours. Roll around a bit in your spine however feels good—maybe side to side, forward and back, or round and round. Breathe really fully and deeply. When you're ready, tuck your toes, take a big inhale, and lift your hips up and back to down dog. Sway a bit here to open up if that feels nice. Pressing into one hand and the other, shifting your hips from side to side, however feels good to you.

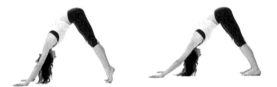

This is a nice opportunity to get out in the room and connect with people. Placing a hand on someone's lower back to help soften is nice.

Take a big inhale and lift up onto your tiptoes. Exhale and soften back. Twice more like that, big inhale and lift up. Soften back and relax. One more time, big inhale and lift. Exhale, soften, and relax.

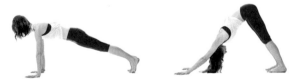

Tuck your chin and round out into your plank, top of your push-up. Hang here for a moment. Sway a bit side to side or forward and back if that feels nice. When you're ready, lift your hips up and back to down dog.

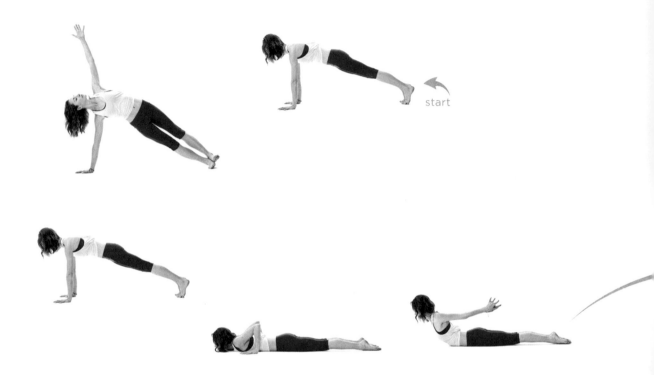

start

Put yourself where people can see you for the side planks. From one side to the other where people are opening up is great. Remember to breathe deeply and move easily in your body as you navigate the room. Let your voice, body, and breath-body connection support you.

You have an opportunity to be in the room supporting with touch in child's pose and down dog.

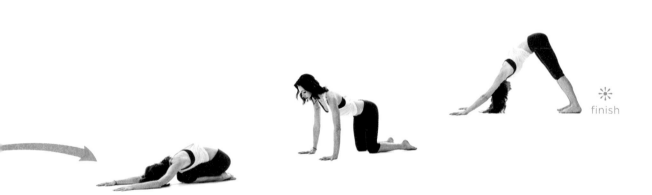

finish

Tuck your chin and round out into plank. Lift your hips up a bit, shift your weight onto your right and the outside edge of your right foot, and open up to a side plank, facing your left side. When you're ready, come back to your middle and open up to your other side. When you're ready, roll back to your plank. Soften your elbows and lower to your belly. Interlace your hands behind you and lift up. Sway a bit here if that feels nice. When you're ready, soften back down. Press your palms on the ground next to your chest and shift your hips back to your heels. Rest here for a moment. When you're ready, come onto all fours, spread your fingers wide, tuck your toes, and take a big inhale to lift up and back to down dog.

FOURTH WAVE

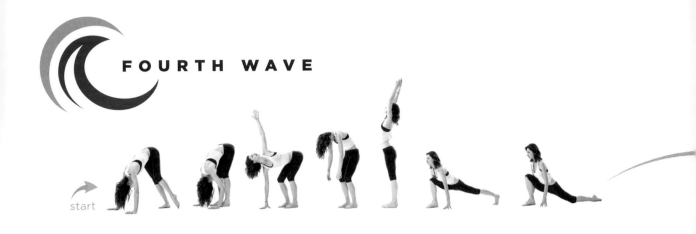

start

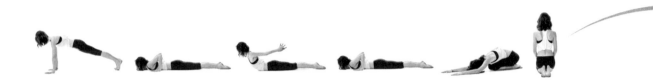

This works either demonstrating and mirroring or being in the room to support with touch or to do the movements alongside people.

Gently walk your feet up to your hands one step at a time. Hands can move too if that feels nice. Once you make it up, soften your torso over your legs. Let your head and neck go. Soften your knees and press your right fingertips on the ground. Take a big inhale and open your body toward your left, opening your left arm up. Easy exhale and soften back through your middle. Press your left fingertips on the ground. Take a big inhale and open up toward your right. Easy exhale and soften back to your middle. Soften your knees and let your head and neck relax.

When you're ready, round up to stand one notch at a time. Once you make it up, take a big inhale and float your arms out and up. Exhale and soften back over your legs. Twice more like that, round up one notch at a time. Once you're up, take a big inhale and lift your arms out and up. Exhale and relax over your legs. One more time, rounding one notch at a time, big inhale reach your arms out and up. Soften back over your legs.

Soften your knees, press your fingertips on the ground, and step your left leg back to your low lunge. Sink your hips here, sway a bit if that feels nice. When you're ready, soften your back knee to the ground and settle here for a moment. Either bring your torso low if that feels nice on your hips, or bring yourself up a bit. Breathe really full and deep. When you're ready, bring your fingertips to the

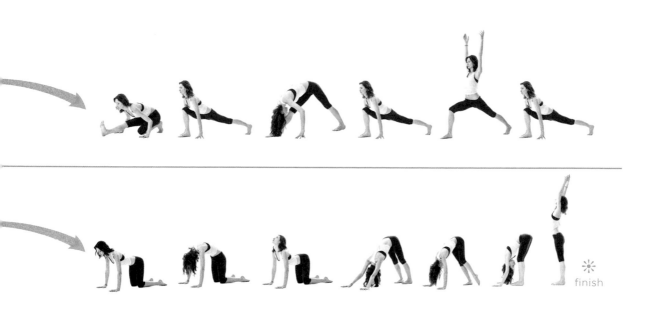

finish

ground, tuck your toes, and shift your hips back to sit on your back heel for your runner's stretch. Relax your torso over your front leg and sway a bit here if that feels nice. When you're ready, crawl yourself back to your low lunge. Press your fingertips to the ground, lift your hips, and relax your torso over your front leg. Sway a bit here if that feels nice. When you're ready, sink back to your low lunge. Press down through your legs and lift up to your high lunge. Soften back to your low lunge, plant your palms, and step back to plank. Soften your elbows and lower to your belly. Interlace your hands behind you and open up for a nice back arch. Sway a bit here if that feels nice. When you're ready, relax back to your belly. Press your palms on the ground and shift back to child's pose. Soften here for a few breaths. When you're ready, round up to sit on your heels. Relax your hands on your thighs, close your eyes, and draw your attention inward. Notice your inhales and exhales as they come and go. When you're ready, gently open your eyes.

   Crawl out onto all fours. Roll around a bit in your spine, staying easy with your breath. When you're ready, tuck your toes, take a big inhale, and lift your hips up and back to down dog. Soften here. When you're ready, walk your feet up toward the top of your mat. Hands can walk too. Come into your standing forward bend. Soften your knees. Relax your head and neck. Settle here for a moment. When you're ready, round up to stand one notch at a time. When you make it up, take a big inhale and float your arms out and up. Exhale and soften back over your legs.

   Repeat the phrase on the other side.

FIFTH WAVE

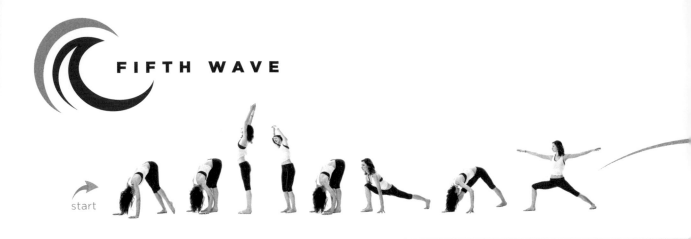

start

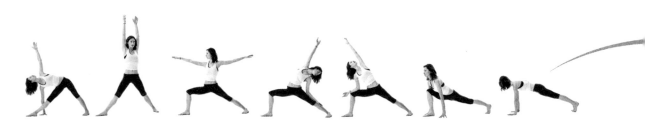

Warrior 2 and movements can be demonstrated on the side, facing the group, or from the front, mirroring and facing the group. Child's pose is another opportunity for touch.

When you're ready, walk your feet up to the top of your mat. Hands can walk too. Soften over your legs to your standing forward bend. Soften your knees. Relax your head and neck. When you're ready, round up to stand one notch at a time. Once you make it up, take a big inhale and float your arms out and up. Grab hold of your left wrist with your right hand. Soften here. Take a big inhale and lift up so much that maybe you run-out-of-up and tip over a bit toward your right. Sway a bit here if that feels nice. When you're ready, bring yourself back to the center and trade hands. Take a big inhale and lift up so much that maybe you tip over toward your left side. Sway here a bit if that feels nice. When you're ready, bring yourself back to center. Take a big inhale and lift everything up. Exhale and soften your torso over your legs.

Soften your knees and step your left foot back to your low lunge. Sink your hips low.

Keeping your fingertips on the ground, take a big inhale and lift your hips up. Relax your torso over your front leg. Relax your head and neck and sway a bit here if that feels nice. Soften your knees, spin your back heel down, press down through your legs, take a big inhale and lift everything up, lifting your hips and arms up. Exhale and soften into your warrior 2 turning your right toes to face your front

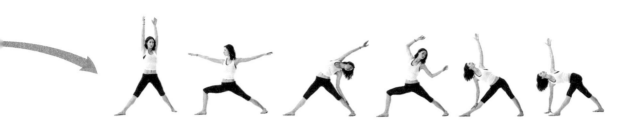

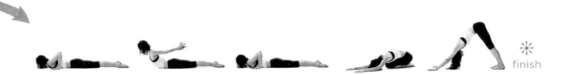

finish

and your left toes slightly in. Open your arms out to your sides. Take a big inhale and lift up a bit. Exhale soften here, sinking your hips, relaxing your head, neck, and shoulders. Take a big inhale and lift up, lifting your hips and arms up. Exhale and soften back to warrior 2. Big inhale, tip back reverse warrior as you lengthen out your front leg. Tip your torso up and over for your triangle, sliding your right hand down your front leg, either landing on your shin or fingertips on the ground. Take a big inhale and open up. Soften your knees, press your left fingertips on the ground, take a big inhale, and open up to your right for your twisted triangle. Soften your knees, press your right fingertips on the ground, take a big inhale and open up to your open triangle. Soften your knees, press down through your legs, take a big inhale and lift up, lifting your hips and arms up. Exhale and soften to warrior 2. Tip back reverse warrior, tip forward to your extended side angle bringing your right forearm to your front thigh and your left arm up and overhead. Roll your body open. When you're ready, come back to your low lunge. Plant your palms on the ground and step back to plank. Soften your elbows and lower to your belly. Interlace your hands behind you and lift up. Sway a bit here if that feels nice. When you're ready, soften back down. Plant your palms on the ground and shift your hips back to sit on your heels for your child's pose. Settle here for a moment. When you're ready, come back onto all fours, spread your fingers wide, tuck your toes, take a big inhale, and lift your hips up and back to down dog.

Repeat on left side, swapping out chair, twisted chair right and left, standing forward bend shoulder release, standing forward bend, for standing side bend right and left.

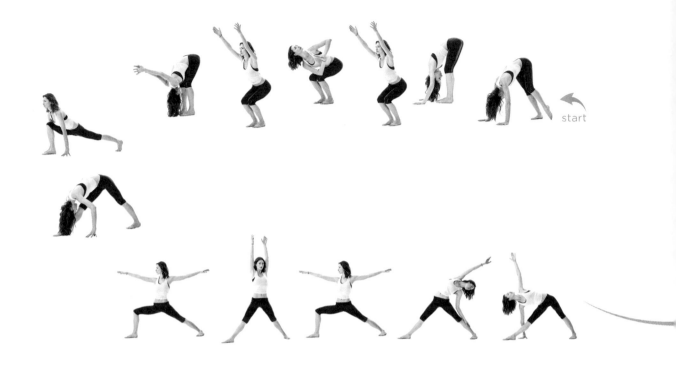

start

You have an opportunity for touch with the standing forward bend. Chair movements are nice to demonstrate facing and mirroring either in front of the whole group or in front of a row, depending on where you are. You could demonstrate the warrior 2 series from the front or the side or be moving throughout the group and demonstrating not with your body full out, but your voice and body connection. This is often a nice choice to be up and stay mobile. You have an opportunity for touch with child's pose and down dog.

When you're ready, walk your feet up to the top of your mat. Hands can walk too. Soften over your legs to your standing forward bend. Soften your knees. Relax your head and neck. When you're ready, sink your hips, take a big inhale, and lift up into chair. Press your palms together and twist to your left, bringing your right elbow outside your left thigh. Take a big inhale and lift back up. Easy exhale and twist toward your right side. Big inhale and lift up. Exhale and dive up and over; interlace your hands behind your back and relax over your legs. Sway a bit here if that feels nice.

Soften your knees and step your right foot back to your low lunge. Sink your hips low. Keeping your fingertips on the ground, take a big inhale and lift your hips up. Relax your torso over your front leg. Relax your head and neck and sway a bit here if that feels nice. Soften your knees, spin your back heel down, press down through your legs, take a big inhale, and lift everything up, lifting your hips and arms up. Exhale and

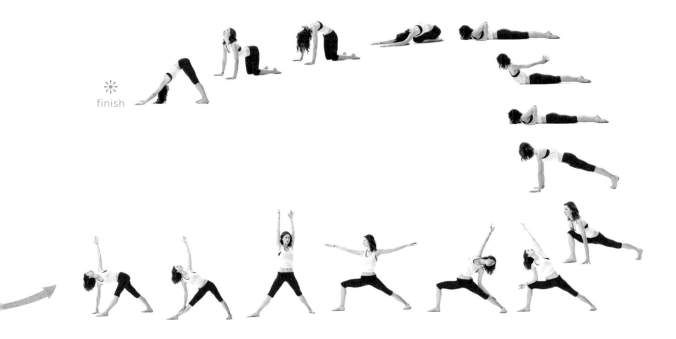

finish

soften into your warrior 2 turning your right toes to face your front and your left toes slightly in. Open your arms out to your sides. Take a big inhale and lift up a bit. Exhale soften here, sinking your hips, relaxing your head, neck, and shoulders. Take a big inhale and lift up, lifting your hips and arms up. Exhale and soften back to warrior 2. Big inhale, tip back reverse warrior as you lengthen out your front leg. Tip your torso up and over for your triangle, sliding your left hand down your front leg either landing on your shin or fingertips on the ground. Take a big inhale and open up. Soften your knees, press your right fingertips on the ground, take a big inhale, and open up to your left for your twisted triangle. Soften your knees, press your left fingertips on the ground, take a big inhale, and open up to your open triangle. Soften your knees, press down through your legs, take a big inhale, and lift up, lifting your hips and arms up. Exhale and soften to warrior 2. Tip back reverse warrior, tip forward to your extended side angle, bringing your left forearm to your front thigh and your right arm up and overhead. Roll your body open. When you're ready, come back to your low lunge. Plant your palms on the ground and step back to plank. Soften your elbows and lower to your belly. Interlace your hands behind you and lift up. Sway a bit here if that feels nice. When you're ready, soften back down. Plant your palms on the ground and shift your hips back to sit on your heels for your child's pose. Settle here for a moment. When you're ready, come back onto all fours, spread your fingers wide, tuck your toes, take a big inhale, and lift your hips up and back to down dog.

SIXTH WAVE

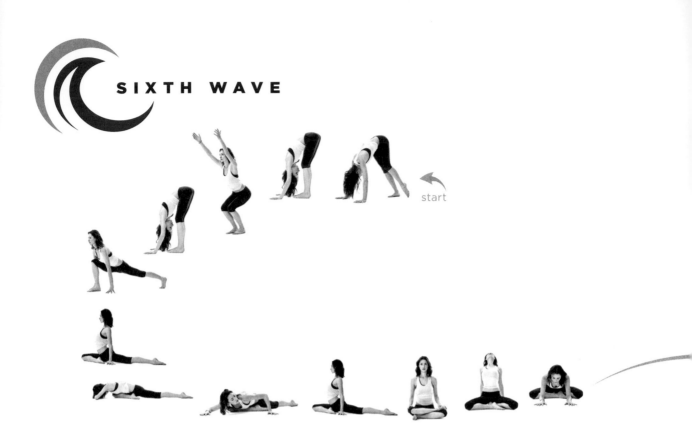

start

This is nice to demonstrate and mirror from the front of the room. Pigeon is an opportunity to make your way to the group for touch and support. You could either come back to the front after pigeon to demonstrate or demonstrate with your voice-body connection and stay in the group to support for the single leg forward bend and down dog.

Walk your feet toward the top of your mat. Hands can walk too. Fold over your legs. Soften your head and neck. Sway a bit here if that feels nice. When you're ready, round up to stand one notch at a time. When you make it up, take a big inhale and float your arms out and up. Exhale and soften over your legs. Soften your knees, press your fingertips on the ground, and step your left leg back to your low lunge. Sink your hips here. When you're ready, move your front foot over toward your left hand and ease your shin on down for your pigeon. Take your time to get comfortable here. Roll around a bit to find a place where you feel a good opening and can breathe really fully. If you feel good here, hang here. If you'd like to take a big inhale and open up, go for that. Either hang here or guide yourself on forward. Crawl around to one side and the other, finding a place where you can settle for a while. (Give several long, deep breaths here.) When you're ready, bring yourself back up. Lean toward your front hip and bring your back leg around, stacking your ankles and knees if that feels

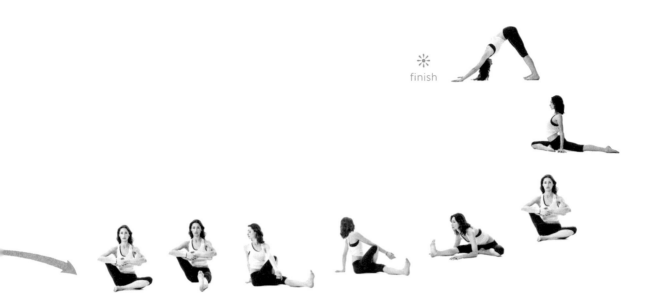

finish

nice or bringing your left leg in front of your right for an easy cross-legged seat. Bring your hands behind you on the ground and lean back and open. Either stay here if this feels nice, or explore your way on forward, crawling around to one side and the other, finding a nice place to settle for a bit. Hang here for a few long, deep breaths. When you're ready, bring yourself back up. Grab hold of your right shin, hugging it toward you. Sway a bit side to side if that feels nice. Lengthen your bottom leg out in front of you. Take a big inhale and give the shin a squeeze; exhale and cross it over your extended leg. Take a big inhale and lift your right arm up; exhale and cross it over your left leg. Bring your left fingertips behind you on the ground. Take a big inhale and lift up tall, exhale and twist around a little farther. Hang here for a few deep breaths. When you're ready, unwind toward the other side. Bring your foot on the ground inside of your extended leg. Relax your hands on the ground beside you. Take a big inhale and open up; exhale and soften over your extend leg. Sway a bit here if that feels nice. When you're ready, bring yourself back up. Hug your shin back in, slide your bottom leg back, and wind your way back to your pigeon. Plant your palms on the ground and make your way back to down dog however feels nice for you. Take your time unwinding this side. Either roll through some cat cows, or stretch one leg up and back, or shift your weight from one side to the other in down dog, or something else that feels good for you. We'll meet in down dog in a bit.

Repeat the phrase on the other side.

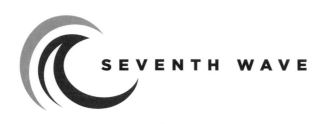

SEVENTH WAVE

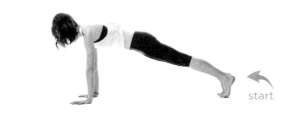

start

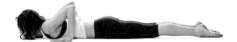

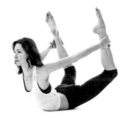

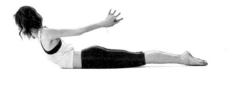

This is nice to demonstrate in the group with your voice and breath-body connection. There is an opportunity when you have people resting between bow and lying on belly for touch, as well as child's pose and down dog.

Tuck your chin and round out to plank. Soften your elbows and lower to your belly. Up to you, either rest here or if you'd like to open up your back a bit, bend your knees, and grab hold of your feet with your hands. Take a big inhale and press your feet into your hands, leaving some room to breathe. If this doesn't feel nice, relax down or interlace your hands behind you and lift up a bit. Sway a bit here if that feels nice. When you're ready,

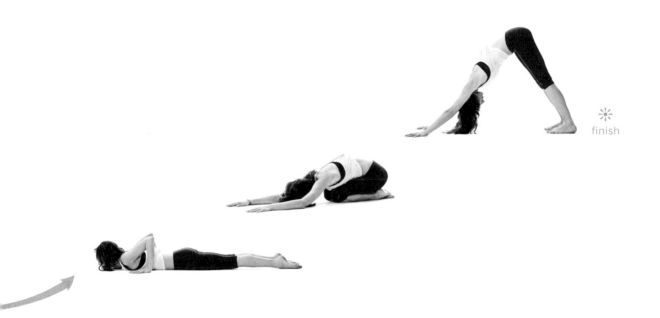

finish

relax down. Turn your head to one side and rest here for a bit. If you'd like to stay here and rest, feel free. If you'd like to go for one more opening, grab hold of your feet or interlace your hands and lift up. Maybe rock a bit side to side or forward and back if that feels nice. When you're ready, relax back down. Turn the other side of your face on the ground and rest for a bit. When you're ready, press your palms on the ground and shift your hips back to your child's pose. Soften here for a bit. When you're ready, come back to all fours, tuck your toes, take a big inhale, and lift your hips up and back to down dog.

EIGHTH WAVE

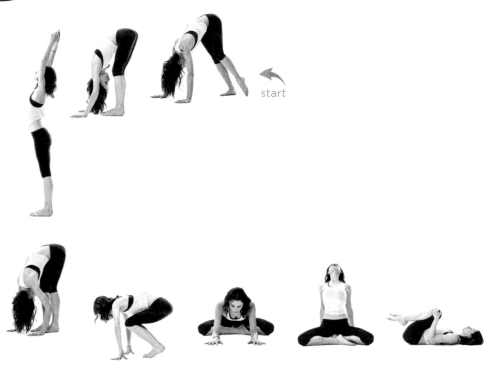

start

Down dog is a nice moment for touch and support, along with standing forward bend. When you make it to rolling up and down and squat and easy forward bend, it's nice to demo in the front, facing and mirroring here. When you guide rolling down, it's nice to get up and be moving around the room so people can hear you and to check if anyone needs help or support.

When you're ready, walk on up to the top of your mat, one step at a time. Hands can walk too. Once you make it up, fold up and over your legs. Soften your knees and sway a bit if that feels nice. Round up to stand one notch at a time. Once you make it up, take a big inhale and float your arms out and up. Exhale and soften up and over your legs.

When you're ready, release your hands, press your palms on the ground, put some weight into your arms, and come into a squat. Roll around a bit here to open up however it feels nice. When you're ready, bring your hands behind you and

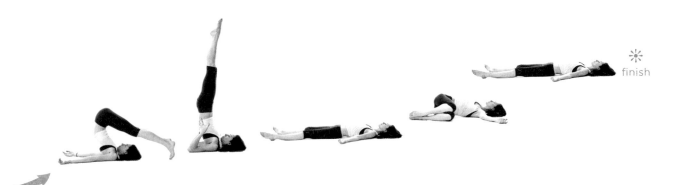

finish

come to sit down easily. Any forward bend that feels nice to you, bringing the bottoms of your feet together, legs apart, or legs forward. Take a big inhale and lean back and open up. Either stay here if this feels nice or guide yourself forward, exploring around to one side and the other, finding a nice place to breathe for a few moments. When you're ready, round on down to your back, carrying your knees along with you. Hug your knees into your chest and either rock side to side to open up or round up and over for your plow. If plow doesn't feel nice on your back and neck, round gently down. If you'd like to evolve your plow into your shoulder stand, bring your palms to support your back and lift your legs up. Wherever you are, breathe really fully and deeply. Feel free to stay there as long as feels nice. When you are ready, ease on back down. Anything else you'd like to roll through before we rest. Maybe a gentle twist side to side. Take your time. When you're ready, stretch out a bit. If there is any tension lingering around, take a big inhale through your nose and long exhale out through your mouth. Twice more just like that. When you're ready, rest here.

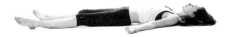

Here you have an opportunity to connect with several people through touch. There's nothing to guide with words here. Moving around the room and supporting people with touch is great.

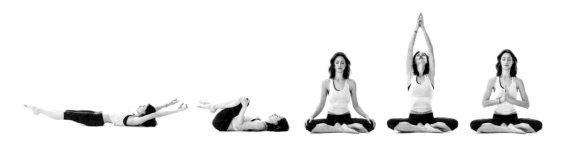

It is great to be in the front of the room, sitting easily, as you guide people to come out of the relaxation and meeting them in easy seated for meditation.

Start to invite some more air back into your body. Roll around your wrists and ankles if that feels nice. Stretch out your arms overhead if that feels nice. When you're ready, hug your knees into your chest and make your way up to sit in the easiest way.

Close your eyes and let your attention drift inward. Take a big inhale and float your arms up and overhead. Press your palms together and bring your thumbs to your heartbeat. Soften here for a moment. Take a big inhale through your nose. Exhale out through your mouth. Twice more like that, big inhale. Long exhale. One more time, big inhale, long exhale. Soften here for a moment.

Namaste and thank you for coming!

CLASS 3: Strala RELAX

THE PURPOSE

The purpose of RELAX is to dissolve physical and mental tension through easygoing movement to enjoy rejuvenation and relaxation.

THE DESCRIPTION

Strala RELAX is a moving flow that releases tension from your body and mind, while resting attention calmly on your breath. You drop the stress and feel revitalized all over!

FIRST WAVE

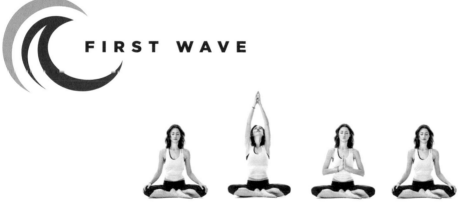

Begin sitting in the front of the room facing the group. Demonstrate along with the group here.

Sit easy, however you can be comfortable. Close your eyes and let your attention rest a bit deeper inward. Take a big inhale and float your arms up and overhead. Press your palms together and bring your thumbs to your heartbeat. Soften here for a moment. All together take a big inhale through your nose. Long exhale out through your mouth. Twice more like that. Big inhale. Long exhale. One more time, big inhale. Long exhale. When you're ready, relax your hands on your thighs.

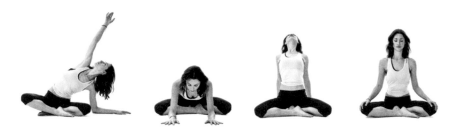

This is great to demonstrate mirroring and facing the group.

Tip over toward your left side, bringing your left forearm to the ground. Open your right arm up and overhead. Sway a bit here if that feels nice. When you're ready, bring yourself back up to the middle. Same thing other side, tipping over, keeping both sides of your waist nice and long.

When you're ready, bring yourself back up through center. Crawl yourself forward a couple steps or a few more if that feels nice. Let your head go. Let your neck go. Sway a bit here if that feels nice. When you're ready, bring yourself back up through center. Bring your fingertips behind you on the ground and lift up. Lift your hips up also if that feels nice. When you're ready, bring yourself back to center. Rest your palms on your thighs, close your eyes, and let your attention drift back inward.

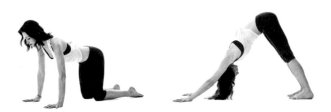

Demonstrate facing and mirroring; sit to one side to come around onto all fours, instead of coming through the middle over your knees. It's a big deal for knee safety not to roll over the knees in this position. What may be easy for you might blow out someone else's knee with a different build or old sports injury. Move gently as you demonstrate.

When you're ready, sit to the side and come around onto all fours. Spread your fingers wide, tuck your toes, take a big inhale, and lift your hips up and back to down dog. Sway a bit here to open up if that feels nice. Pressing into one hand and then the other, shifting your hips from side to side, however feels good to you.

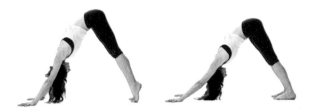

This is a nice opportunity to get out in the room and connect with people. Placing a hand on someone's lower back to help soften is nice.

Take a big inhale and lift up onto your tiptoes. Exhale and soften back. Twice more like that, big inhale and lift up. Soften back and relax. One more time, big inhale and lift. Exhale, soften, and relax.

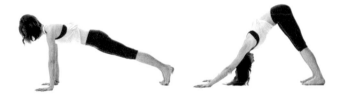

Remember to breathe deeply and move easily in your body as you navigate the room. Let your voice, body, and breath-body connection support you.

Tuck your chin and round out into your plank, the top of your push-up. Hang here for a moment. Sway a bit side to side or forward and back if that feels nice. When you're ready, lift your hips up and back to down dog.

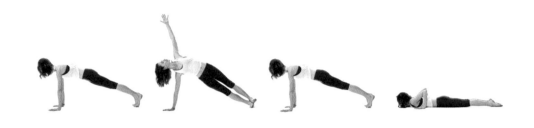

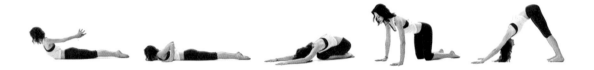

Put yourself where people can see you for the side planks. From one side to the other where people are opening up is great, demonstrating with your voice-body connection but on your feet so you can move easily around the room. Here you have an opportunity to be in the room supporting with touch in child's pose and down dog.

Tuck your chin and round out into plank. Lift your hips up a bit, shift your weight onto your right and the outside edge of your right foot, and open up to a side plank, facing your left side. When you're ready, come back to your middle and open up to your other side. When you're ready, roll back to your plank. Soften your elbows and lower to your belly. Interlace your hands behind you and lift up. Sway a bit here if that feels nice. When you're ready, soften back down. Press your palms on the ground next to your chest and shift your hips back to your heels. Rest here for a moment. When you're ready, come onto all fours, spread your fingers wide, tuck your toes, and take a big inhale to lift up and back to down dog.

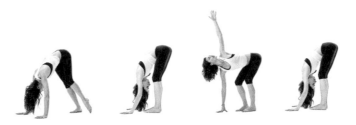

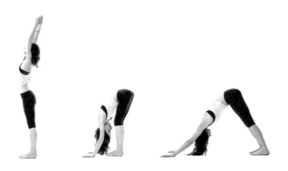

This works either demonstrating and mirroring or being in the room to support with touch or to do the movements alongside people.

Gently walk your feet up to your hands one step at a time. Hands can move too if that feels nice. Once you make it up, soften your torso over your legs. Let your head and neck go. Soften your knees and press your right fingertips on the ground. Take a big inhale and open your body toward your left, opening your left arm up. Easy exhale and soften back through your middle. Press your left fingertips on the ground. Take a big inhale and open up toward your right. Easy exhale and soften back to your middle. Soften your knees and let your head and neck relax.

When you're ready, round up to stand one notch at a time. Once you make it up, take a big inhale and float your arms out and up. Exhale and soften back over your legs. Twice more like that, round up one notch at a time. Once you're up, take a big inhale and lift your arms out and up. Exhale and relax over your legs. One more time, rounding one notch at a time, big inhale reach your arms out and up. Soften back over your legs. Soften your knees, plant your palms on the ground, and make your way back to down dog.

SECOND WAVE

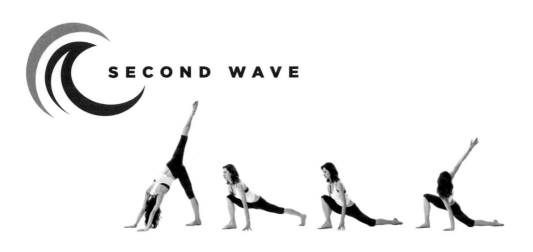

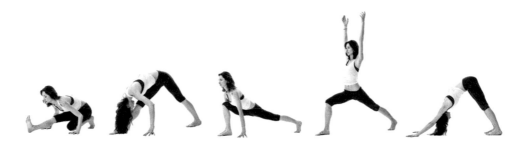

After the down dog split, this phrase, along with most standing movement phrases that move from side to side, is nice to demo and mirror while facing the group.

Take a big inhale and lift your right leg up and back to down dog split. Open your hips and shoulders if that feels nice. Step your foot on through for low lunge. Soften here. Ease your back knee down and open up a bit here. Press your left fingertips on the ground, take a big inhale, and open up toward your right, opening your right arm up. Soften and bring both fingertips to the ground and sink your hips back toward your back heel for your runner's stretch. Relax your torso over your front leg. Sway a bit here if that feels nice. When you're ready, crawl yourself back to your low lunge, press down through your legs, take a big inhale, and lift up to your high lunge. Exhale and soften back down. Plant your palms on the ground and make your way back to down dog.

Repeat the phrase on the other side.

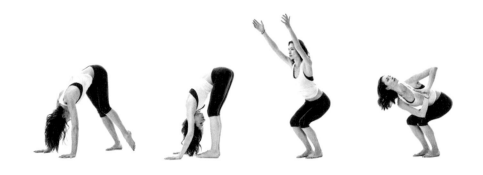

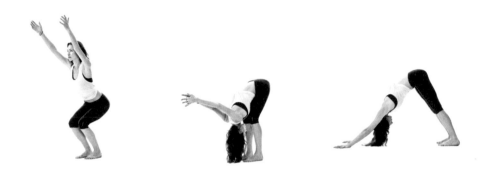

This is a nice place to mirror and demo while facing the group.

When you're ready, walk on up to the top of your mat. Hands can walk too if that feels nice. Fold over your legs. Soften your knees. Sway a bit here if you'd like. When you're ready, sink your hips, take a big inhale, and lift up into chair. Press your palms together and twist to your left, bringing your right elbow outside your left thigh. Take a big inhale and lift back up. Easy exhale and twist toward your opposite side. Big inhale and lift up. Exhale and dive up and over, interlacing your hands behind your back and relaxing over your legs. Sway a bit here if that feels nice. When you're ready, release your hands, press your palms on the ground, soften your knees, and make your way back to down dog.

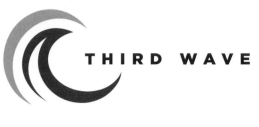

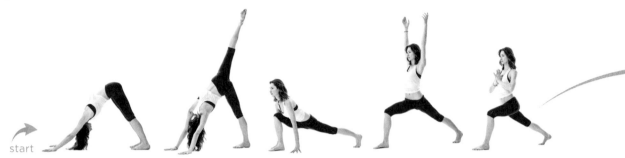

start

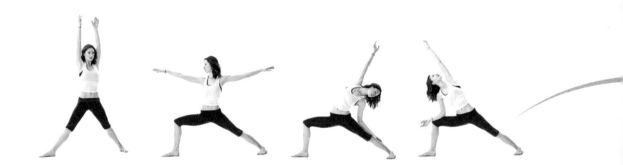

These longer standing movement phrases are nice to demonstrate mirroring and facing the group. There is no need to demonstrate a down dog split while you are speaking. People can't see or hear you. Take the opportunity when people are in down dog to touch and make contact with someone. You can support the down dog split with your voice and body, moving through the room. You can meet the group in the front at low lunge and pick up your mirroring from there.

Soften in your down dog. Sway a bit here to keep things easy and gentle in your body. Take a big inhale and lift your right leg up and back to down dog split. Open your hips and shoulders if that feels nice. Step your foot between your hands to low lunge. Press down through your legs and lift up to your high lunge. Press your palms together and bring your thumbs to your heartbeat. Take a big inhale and lift; exhale and twist toward your left, bringing your right elbow outside your

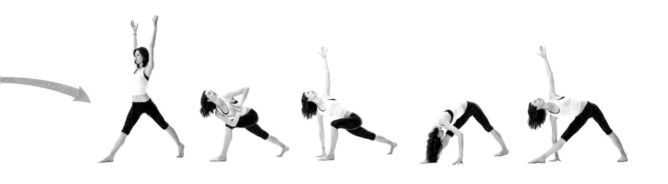

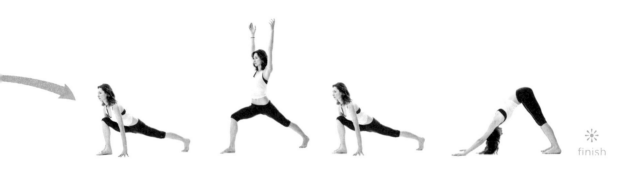

finish

left thigh. Open up your arms, bringing your right fingertips to the ground for support. Take a big inhale, and open up toward your left. When you're ready, bring both fingertips to the ground on either side of your front foot, lift your hips, and relax your torso over your front leg. Sway a bit here if that feels nice. Spin your back heel to the ground and open up to your body to your left side for your triangle. Soften through your knees, press down through your legs, and lift everything up, lifting your hips and raising your arms up overhead, soften into your warrior 2. Tip back reverse. Tip up and over to your extended side angle, pressing your forearm to your thigh. Roll your body open. Bring your fingertips to the ground on either side of your front foot coming into your low lunge. Press down through your legs, take a big inhale, and lift up to your high lunge. Exhale back to your low lunge, plant your palms, and make your way back to down dog.

Repeat the phrase on the other side.

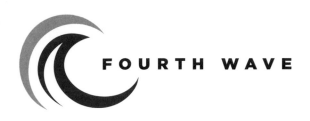

FOURTH WAVE

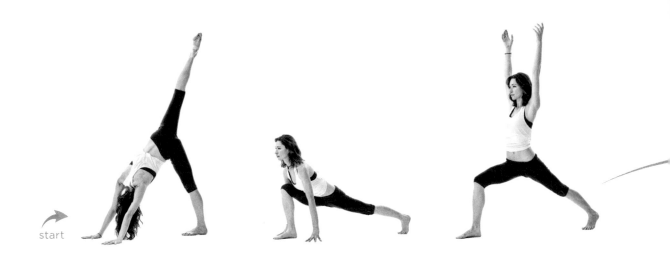

start

This is nice to be in the mix of the group, demonstrating with your breath and voice to support the flow and not full out with the movements.

Take a big inhale and lift your right leg up and back to down dog split. Open your hips and shoulders if that feels nice. Step it on through to low lunge. Press down through your legs and lift up to high lunge. Exhale and soften back down, press your palms on the ground, and make your way back to down dog.

Take a big inhale and lift your right leg up and back to down dog split. Open your hips and shoulders if that feels nice. Step it on through to low lunge. Press down through your legs and lift up to high lunge. Exhale and soften back down, press your palms on the ground, and make your way back to down dog.

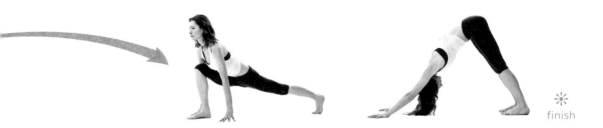

finish

One more round like that.

Take a big inhale and lift your right leg up and back to down dog split. Open your hips and shoulders if that feels nice. Step it on through to low lunge. Press down through your legs and lift up to high lunge. Exhale and soften back down, press your palms on the ground, and make your way back to down dog.

Take a big inhale and lift your right leg up and back down to dog split. Open your hips and shoulders if that feels nice. Step it on through to low lunge. Press down through your legs and lift up to high lunge. Exhale and soften back down, press your palms on the ground, and make your way back to down dog.

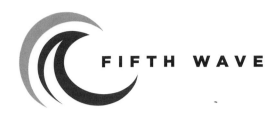

FIFTH WAVE

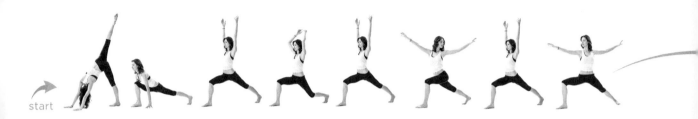

start

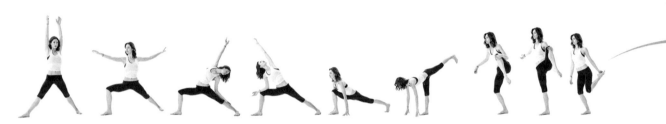

**This phrase is nice to demonstrate facing the group and mirroring.
You could make your way to the side to demonstrate for the warrior 2
movements and back up front for rolling up on through to dancer and
tree on through high and low lunge. You have an opportunity for touch
with down dog.**

Take a big inhale and lift your right leg up and back to down dog split. Open
your hips and shoulders if that feels nice. Step it on through to low lunge. Press down
through your legs and lift up to high lunge. Exhale and soften here. Inhale lift to high
lunge. Exhale twist toward your left, with your arms open wide. Inhale back up to high
lunge. Twice more like that, easy exhale twist and open, big inhale back up. One more
time, easy exhale twist, big inhale back up, and open to warrior 2. Soften here. Relax
your head, neck, and shoulders. Take a big inhale and lift up. Lift your hips and arms
up. Exhale and soften back to warrior 2. Big inhale and lift up. Exhale and soften back.
One more time, inhale and fill up. Exhale and settle back. Tip back reverse. Lengthen
your front leg. Tip up and over toward your triangle, sliding your right hand down your
front thigh, either landing on your shin or fingertips on the ground. Open up here.
Soften your knees, press your left fingertips on the ground, and open up toward your
right for your twisted triangle. Soften your knees, press your right fingertips on the
ground, and open up to your open triangle. Soften your knees, press down through
your legs, and lift up, lifting your hips and arms up. Soften back to warrior 2. Tip back

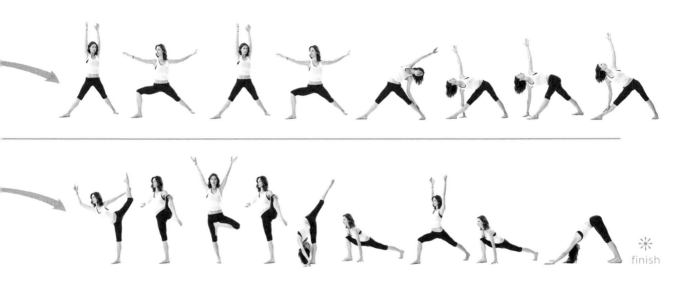

finish

reverse. Tip up and over for your extended side angle. Press your right forearm on your thigh and your left arm up and over your head. Roll your body open.

When you're ready, bring your fingertips to the ground and come into your low lunge. Sink your hips and sway a bit if that feels nice. Lift your hips, soften your knees, crawl your fingertips out in front of you, and float your back leg up for your warrior 3. Soften your knees and round up to stand, hugging your left shin along with you. Roll around in your hips here if that feels nice. When you're ready, drop your knee toward the ground and catch hold of your foot behind you. Soften here for a moment. Take a big inhale and gently press your foot into your hand and reach your opposite arm up for your dancer. Soften out of this and hug your shin for a squeeze. Roll around in your hips if that feels nice. When you're ready open up into your tree, pressing your foot into your thigh or resting your toes on the ground, foot into your ankle, however is best for your balance. Open your arms up and settle here for a moment. Soften and sway a bit in the breeze if that feels nice. When you're ready, hug your shin back into your chest, take a big inhale and lift up, exhale dive up and over your leg, bringing your fingertips to the ground. Relax your head and neck for your standing split. Soften your knees and step your top leg back for low lunge. Press down through your legs, take a big inhale, and lift up to high lunge. Exhale back down, plant your palms, and make your way back to down dog.

Repeat the phrase on the other side.

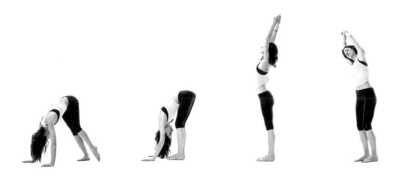

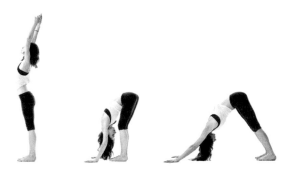

Standing forward bend is a nice moment to connect with someone for support on the lower back. Demonstrating the side stretch is useful mirroring, and then get back to the group to connect with someone on down dog.

When you're ready, walk your feet up to the top of your mat. Hands can walk too if that feels nice. When you make it up, fold up and over your legs. Relax your head and neck and soften your knees if that feels nice. When you're ready, round up to stand one notch at a time. Once you make it up, float your arms out and up overhead. Grab hold of your left wrist with your right hand. Soften here. Take a big inhale and lift up, so much that maybe you run-out-of-up and tip over a bit toward your right side. Hang here for a bit, rolling around however it feels nice. When you're ready, come back to center and go for the other side, grabbing hold of your right wrist with your left hand. Soften here. Take a big inhale and lift up and over toward your left. Hang here for a few big breaths. When you're ready, come back to center. Take a big inhale and open up. Exhale and soften up and over your legs to your standing forward bend. Soften your knees, plant your palms on the ground, and make your way back to down dog.

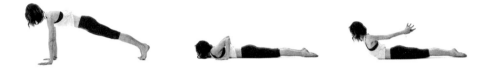

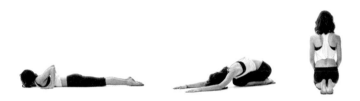

Rolling out to plank and the back arch can be nice to demonstrate showing the movements with your body while you are still standing and moving around the room. It's nice to stay on your feet when you're about to have two great chances to connect with touch coming up: child's pose and down dog. It can be too hectic if you are demonstrating full out and then jumping up quickly to touch someone in child's pose. A fast movement you do as a Guide that you don't mean as an instruction can be confused with an instruction. Moving gracefully and gradually will allow people to connect what you are doing and what you are saying seamlessly.

When you're ready, tuck your chin and round out to plank. Soften your elbows and lower to your belly. Interlace your hands behind you, take a big inhale, and open up the front of your body. Sway a bit here if that feels nice. When you're ready, soften back to your belly and relax. Press your palms on the ground and bring your hips to your heels and rest in child's pose. Soften here for a few big breaths. When you're ready, bring yourself up to sit on your heels.

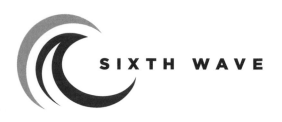

SIXTH WAVE

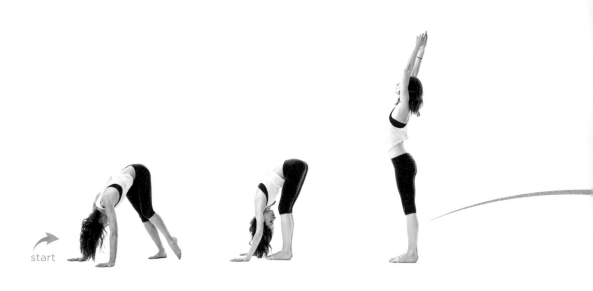

start

Part of this movement phrase is a time period for moving and breathing in any way that feels good. During this time, it's nice to walk people through the first sun salutation. You can do this while moving around the room. If you notice anyone in child's pose or pigeon or down dog during this free time, it can be nice to connect with them through touch. If everyone is moving quite a bit, it makes sense to not interfere and hang on the side or the back of the room for a few moments. Often people will take this time to work on handstands or something more challenging, and it's nice to offer support when appropriate. The main thing is you place yourself where you feel comfortable so people feel free to move and explore. Give people enough time to move freely, and when you have everyone meet in child's pose, you have another opportunity for support.

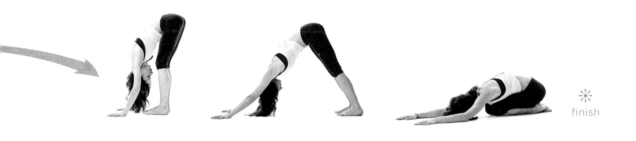

finish

When you're ready, take an easy walk up to the top of your mat. Once you make it up, fold up and over your legs. Soften here for a moment. When you're ready, round up to stand one notch at a time. Once you make it up, take a big inhale and float your arms out and up. Exhale and soften up and over your legs. Soften your knees, plant your palms, and make your way back to down dog however feels great for you. We'll move and breathe for a while here. If you'd like to stay with a simple sun salutation, something coming up and something coming back, great. If you'd like to rest in child's pose, that's great too, or anything else in between. Let the next few moments be an easygoing moving meditation. If you notice your attention drifting, see if you can guide your attention inward, right back to your breath. We'll stay with this for a little while. Stay easy and enjoy the ride.

When you're ready, we'll meet in a child's pose.

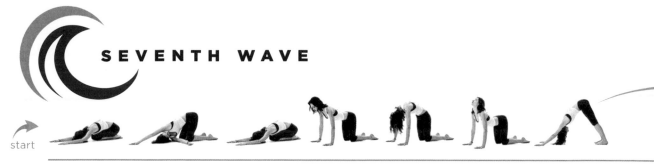

SEVENTH WAVE

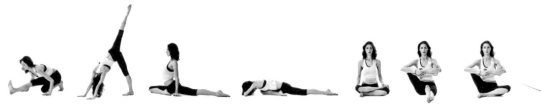

Child's pose is a nice place to connect with people with touch. Warrior 1 series is nice to demonstrate and mirror. Generally you take several breaths in pigeon and ankle to knee, so these are great places to connect with people, and you can usually get to more than one person for each position. The seated twists and unwinding back to pigeon are nice to demonstrate and mirror for clarity. When it comes to down dog, you have another great opportunity to connect through touch.

Rest in child's pose for a few deep breaths. When you're ready, lift up a bit and thread your right arm under your left arm, resting your right shoulder on the ground. If it feels nice to lift your hips up a bit, roll around and find a great spot, go for it. Once you find a great spot, hang here for a few deep breaths. When you're ready, come back to your child's pose in the center and rest for a bit. When you're ready, lift up your hips a bit and thread your left arm under your right arm, resting your right shoulder on the ground. Roll around a bit here to find a great spot, breathing really big and fully and deeply.

When you're ready, come back to the center and rest in child's pose for a few breaths. When you're ready, come onto all fours and roll around a bit in your spine however it feels nice. Maybe cat and cow, or side to side, or round and round—whatever feels good for you. When you're ready, tuck your toes, take a big inhale, and lift up and back to down dog. Soften here for a bit.

When you're ready, take a big inhale and lift your right leg up and back to down dog split. Open your hips and belly if that feels nice. Exhale and step your foot on through to low lunge. Ground your back heel down, so both feet are planted, press down through your legs, and lift up to warrior 1. Settle here for a bit, rolling around in your hips to find a good place. Take a few breaths here. When you're ready, drop your hands behind you, interlace them together, take a big inhale, and lift your chest up. Exhale and fold up and over inside your front leg. Press down through your legs, take a big inhale, and lift up. Exhale and fold up and over your leg.

When you're ready, relax your hands on the ground inside your front foot. Come onto your back toes and move your front foot over to your right side of your mat. Ease your back knee down to the ground and soften here. If you feel good upright, stay here. If it feels nicer to soften your elbows and come onto one or both forearms, go for that, moving softly so you can find a great place. If you feel great in your hips, feel free to stay here;

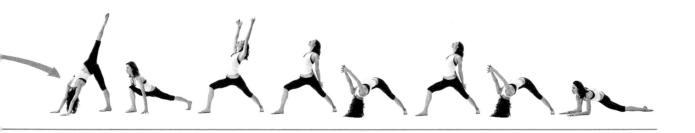

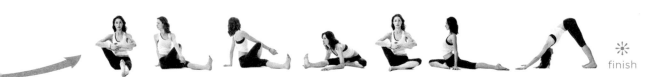

※ finish

if you'd like to get in to your hamstrings, either start to bring your hips back toward your back heel for your runner's stretch, or slide your front leg out to the side a bit or straight forward and back a bit. Move easily so you can find a place where you feel a nice opening but you can still breathe really fully and deeply. We'll hang here for a few deep breaths.

When you're ready, we'll meet up in a down dog split. Either slide your front foot straight back, or lean into your hip, take your time, and roll around to lift your right leg to down dog split. Take a big inhale and open your hips and shoulders if that feels nice. Exhale and soften into your pigeon, bringing your right shin forward and resting on your hip. Take some time to get comfortable here. It's up to you if you'd like to take a big inhale, lean back, and stay upright. If you'd like to crawl yourself forward, maybe explore around to one side and the other to find a great place, go for that. We'll hang here for a few long, deep breaths. If you feel great here, feel free to stay here. If you're ready to come on up, gently bring yourself up. Maybe twist around to one side and the other to open up a bit. Lean into your front hip, and bring your back leg around. If it feels nice to stack your ankles and knees on top of each other, go for that. If that doesn't feel nice, bring your left shin in front of your right to sit easy. Up to you. Either stay upright, lean back, and take a big inhale, or crawl on forward, exploring around to one side and the other to find a good place to rest for a bit. When you're ready, bring yourself on up.

Grab hold of your top shin, hugging it into your chest. Take a big inhale to sit up tall, and slide your bottom leg out in front of you. Give your shin a squeeze as you inhale. Exhale and place your left foot outside your extended leg. Take a big inhale and lift your right arm up. Exhale and cross your arm over your left leg, pressing your left fingertips on the ground behind you. Take a big inhale and lift up tall. Exhale and twist around a little farther. Breathing through that a few times on your own. When you're ready, unwind and twist around to your other side. When you're ready, bring yourself back around toward your front. Bring your left foot on the ground so the bottom of your foot faces toward your thigh. Take a big inhale and sit up tall. Exhale and fold up and over your leg. Sway a bit here if that feels nice. When you're ready, bring yourself back up and we'll unwind to your pigeon. Hug your top shin in toward your chest, slide your bottom leg in, and unwind back to your pigeon. Plant your palms on the ground and make your way back to down dog however feels nice for you.

Repeat the phrase on the other side, from down dog split to warrior 1.

EIGHTH WAVE

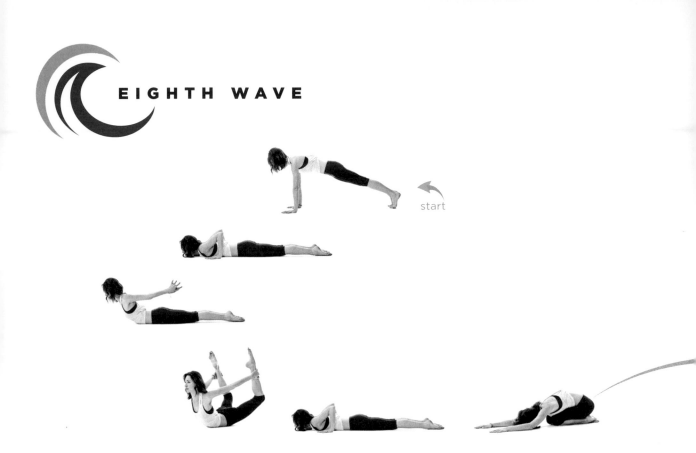

start

Plank and back opener are good times to move around the room demonstrating while you walk. It's nice to stay movable so you can connect with people through touch when they relax on their bellies and in child's pose. Coming to the front of the room to demonstrate the meditation and breathing techniques and doing that along with everyone is sensible to anchor the room. It's also nice to take a few minutes for this breathing section. Use your judgment for the appropriate timing for your group.

When you're ready, tuck your chin and round out to your plank. Soften your elbows and lower to your belly. We'll open up your back a bit. Up to you, either stay here and relax, or interlace your hands behind you and open up a bit. If you'd rather go for a bow pose, bend your knees, catch your feet behind you, and gently press your feet into your hands, leaving some room to breathe fully. When you're ready, soften and relax for a bit. Either stay here or go for one more round. Soften and relax for a bit whenever feels good. When you're ready, press your palms

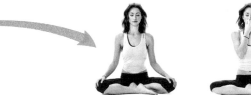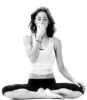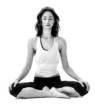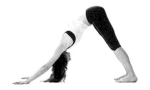

finish

on the ground and shift your hips back to rest in child's pose for a few big, deep breaths. When you're ready, come up to sit however you can be comfortable. We'll breathe here for a bit.

If you'd like to close your eyes, relax your hands on your thighs and breathe, that's great. If you'd like to go for some alternate nostril breathing to calm things even more, that's what we'll be doing next. If this is new for you, it's simple. Take your first two fingers of your right hand like you're saying "peace," curl those fingers in so you have your ring finger and your thumb up, just enough room for your nose in between. Close your eyes and close your left nostril with your ring finger. Take a big inhale up through your right nostril. Then close your right nostril with your thumb and hold the air in for a moment. When you're ready, release your left nostril and breathe out. Repeat this a few times on your own. If you're breathing naturally, continue to breathe naturally. If you notice your attention drifting, guide your attention back to your breath. We'll stay with this for a while. When you're ready, relax your hands on your thighs and come back to your breath. Gently make your way back to down dog when you feel ready.

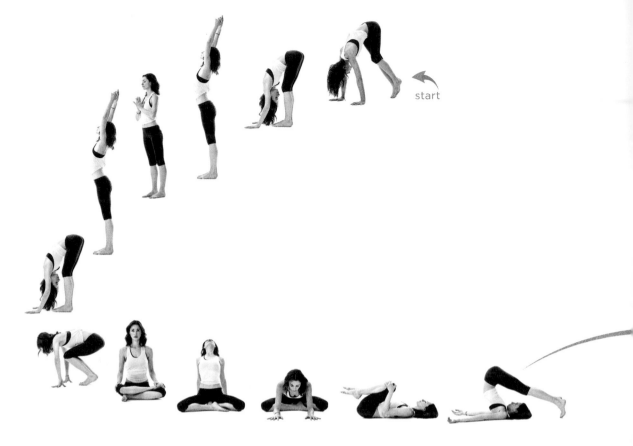

start

Down dog is a great place again to connect with someone through touch. Making your way back to the front of the room to demonstrate the roll up and thumbs to heartbeat is nice for bringing everyone together for a quiet moment, similar to the beginning and end thumbs to heartbeat moment. It's nice to demonstrate options for forward bends, and then you can gracefully get up to support any final movements before relaxation.

When you're ready, walk on up to the top of your mat, one step at a time. Hands can walk too. Once you make it up, fold up and over your legs. Soften your knees and sway a bit if that feels nice. Round up to stand one notch at a time. Once you make it up, take a big inhale and float your arms out and up. Bring your palms together and press your thumbs to your heartbeat. Soften here for a moment. When you're ready, take a big inhale and lift your arms up. Exhale and soften up and over your legs.

When you're ready, press your palms on the ground, put some weight into your arms, and come into a squat. Roll around a bit here to open up however it

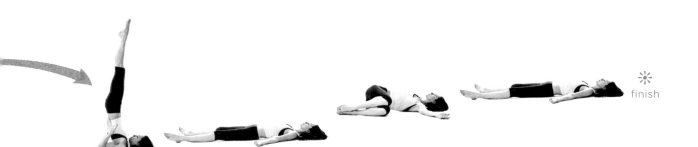

finish

feels nice. When you're ready, bring your hands behind you and come to sit down easily. Do any forward bend that feels nice to you, either bringing the bottoms of your feet together, legs apart, or legs forward. Take a big inhale and lean back and open up. Either stay here if this feels nice or guide yourself forward, exploring around to one side and the other, finding a nice place to breathe for a few moments. When you're ready, round on down to your back, carrying your knees along with you. Hug your knees into your chest and either rock side to side to open up, or round up and over for your plow. If plow doesn't feel nice on your back and neck, round gently down. If you'd like to evolve your plow into your shoulder stand, bring your palms to support your back and lift your legs up. Wherever you are, breathe really fully and deeply. Feel free to stay there as long as feels nice. When you are ready, ease on back down. Anything else you'd like to roll through before we rest. Maybe a gentle twist side to side. Take your time. When you're ready, stretch out a bit. If there is any tension lingering around, take a big inhale through your nose and long exhale out through your mouth. Twice more just like that. When you're ready, rest here.

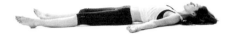

Here you have an opportunity to connect with several people through touch. There's nothing to guide with words here. Moving around the room, supporting people with touch, is great.

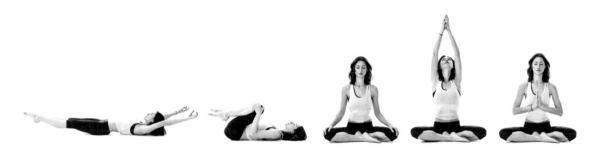

It's great to be in the front of the room, sitting easily, as you guide people to come out of the relaxation and meet them in easy seated for meditation.

Start to invite some more air back into your body. Roll around your wrists and ankles if that feels nice. Stretch out your arms overhead if that feels nice. When you're ready, hug your knees into your chest, and make your way up to sit in the easiest way.

Close your eyes and let your attention drift inward. Take a big inhale and float your arms up and overhead. Press your palms together and bring your thumbs to your heartbeat. Soften here for a moment. Take a big inhale through your nose. Exhale out through your mouth. Twice more like that, big inhale. Long exhale. One more time, big inhale, long exhale. Soften here for a moment.

Namaste and thank you for coming!

CLASS 4: Strala ENERGIZE

THE PURPOSE

The purpose of ENERGIZE is to build body awareness and a healthy amount of strength and mobility and energize the body and mind. ENERGIZE is a great class to practice regularly to build and maintain a healthy and strong body and calm and focused mind.

THE DESCRIPTION

Strala ENERGIZE is a moving flow that invigorates your body and mind while resting attention calmly on your breath. You'll feel awake, energized, and supercreative!

FIRST WAVE

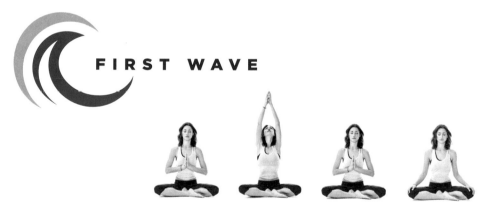

Begin sitting in the front of the room facing the group. Demonstrate along with the group here.

Sit easy, however you can be comfortable. Close your eyes and let your attention rest a bit deeper inward. Take a big inhale and float your arms up and overhead. Press your palms together and bring your thumbs to your heartbeat. Soften here for a moment. All together take a big inhale through your nose. Long exhale out through your mouth. Twice more like that. Big inhale. Long exhale. One more time, big inhale. Long exhale. When you're ready, relax your hands on your thighs.

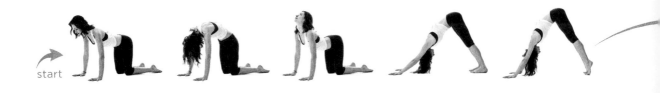

start

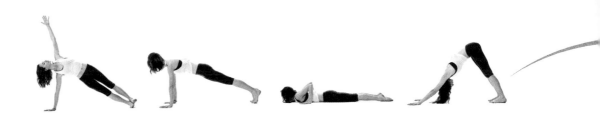

The cat cow is nice to demo, and then you can stand up and get into the group to make contact for down dog. For side planks, standing is also best so that you are able to move freely around the room and can be on the side where people can see and hear you. It's nice to be in the front to demo and mirror the roll up and roll down phrase to encourage the fullness of breath and movement with your own voice and breath-body connection.

Pick a side to lean off to and bring your legs around behind you, coming onto all fours. Roll around a bit here to open up. When you're ready, tuck your toes, take a big inhale, and lift up and back to down dog. Settle here for a bit. Take a big inhale and lift up on to your tiptoes. Exhale, soften back, and relax. Twice more like that. Big inhale lift up. Exhale, soften, and relax. One more time, big inhale and lift. Exhale, soften, and relax.

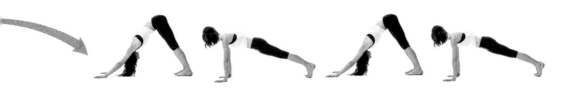

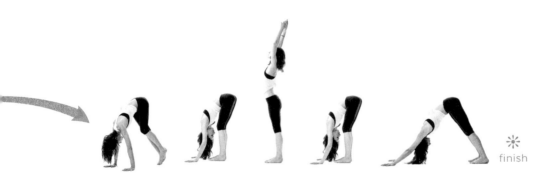

※ finish

   Tuck your chin and round out to your plank. Settle here for a moment. Sway a bit side to side or forward and back to open up a bit. When you're ready, lift your hips up and back to down dog. Tuck your chin and round out to your plank. Lift your hips and shift onto your right side. Take a big inhale and open up to your left. When you're ready, come back to your center. Shift onto your left side. Take a big inhale and open up to your right. When you're ready, come back to center. Soften your elbows and lower to your belly. Press right up and back to down dog.

   Take a walk up to the top of your mat. Hands can walk too. Once you make it up, fold up and over your legs. Relax your head and neck. Sway a bit here if that feels nice. When you're ready, round up to stand one notch at a time. Once you make it up, take a big inhale and float your arms out and up. Exhale and soften up and over your legs. Twice more like that, rounding up, big inhale; take up all the room. Exhale up and over your legs. Once more time, rounding up one notch at a time. Take a big inhale and fill up. Exhale and soften up and over your legs. Soften your knees, plant your palms, and make your way back to down dog however feels great for you.

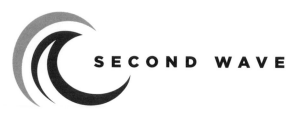

SECOND WAVE

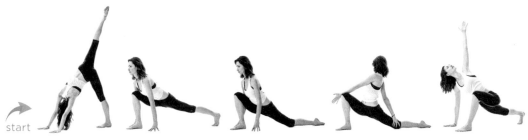

start

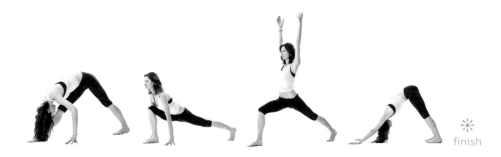

finish

Support people through the down dog split with your voice and breath-body connection, and then head to the front of the room and begin to face and mirror the phrase starting with low lunge. Down dog is a great time to gracefully support people with touch.

Take a big inhale and lift your right leg up and back to down dog split. Open your hips and shoulders if that feels nice. Step your foot on through to low lunge. Soften here. When you're ready, ease your back knee down. If it feels nice to bring your torso down inside your leg, go for that. If it feels nicer to open up, that's great too. When you're ready, bring your left fingertips to the ground, take a big inhale, and open to your right. Soften back to center. Press your right fingertips down, take a big inhale, and open to your left. Come back to center, press both fingertips on the ground, take a big inhale, lift your hips up, and relax your torso over your front leg. Soften your knees and relax your head and neck. When you're ready, sink your hips back to low lunge. Press down through your legs, take a big inhale, and lift up to high lunge. Exhale back down and make your way to down dog however feels great for you.

Repeat the phrase on the other side.

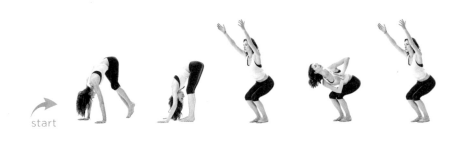

start

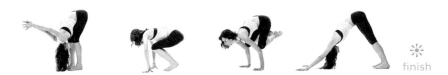

finish

Crow is great to demo either in the front of the room or alongside anyone who is having trouble relaxing through the movement. Come alongside individuals and show them with your demonstration how they can easily rock forward and back with their breath. Usually what happens is they are jumping or stopping their movement in the pose, which stops the ability for the movement to happen effectively. Often it's as simple as showing them they can look more forward, and that is the key for them to be able to accomplish this move with ease. Make sure to show the *process* in your own body, much more than any finished position.

When you're ready, take a walk up to the top of your mat. Hands can walk too. Once you get there, fold up and over your legs. Soften your knees a bit here and relax your head and neck. When you're ready, sink your hips, take a big inhale, and lift up to your chair. Bring your palms together and twist toward your left. Take a big inhale back to your chair. Exhale and twist toward your right. Big inhale back to your chair. Exhale, fold up and over your legs, and interlace your hands behind you for a shoulder release. Soften your knees and sway a bit here if that feels nice. Relax your head and neck. When you're ready, bring your hands to the ground in front of you. Bring some weight into your arms and sink your hips to your squat. Sway a bit here to open up your hips and belly if that feels nice. Up to you, either stay with this, or if you want to go for your crow, plant your palms on the ground in front of you, take a big inhale, lean forward, and look forward. Exhale, soften back, and relax. Go for this a few times with your breath. As you inhale squeeze your knees around your arms, looking forward and leaning forward. Exhale, soften back, and relax. Roll through this a few times with your breath, and when you're ready, make your way back to down dog, however feels great for you.

THIRD WAVE

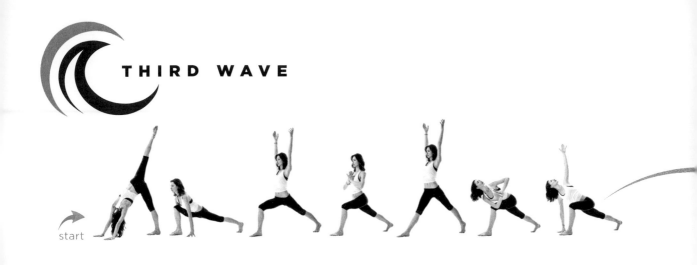

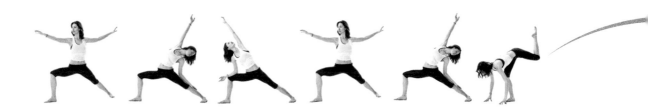

start

After the down dog split, this phrase is nice to demonstrate facing and mirroring. When you get to warrior 2, it's nice to demonstrate on the side where people can see and hear you and make your way back up to the front for the balance movements. Down dog is your opportunity to make contact through touch and support.

Take a big inhale and float your right leg up and back to down dog split. Open your hips and shoulders if that feels nice. Exhale and step your foot between your hands for low lunge. Press down through your legs, take a big inhale, and lift up to high lunge. Bring your palms together and bring your thumbs to your heartbeat. Soften here. Take a big inhale lift. Exhale and twist toward your left. Either stay here or open your arms for a little more support, bringing your right fingertips to the ground and your left arm up, opening to your left. When you're ready, bring both fingertips to the ground on either side of your front foot. Take a big inhale and lift your hips up and relax your torso over your front leg. Sway a bit here if that feels nice. Soften your knees and crawl yourself out to your warrior 3, letting your back leg float up. Soften your knees, press your left fingertips to the ground,

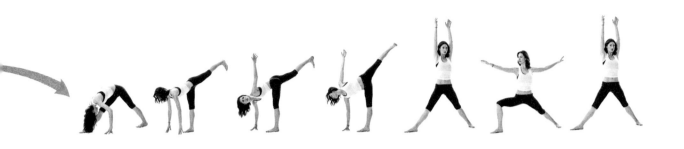

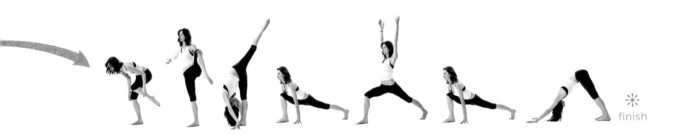

finish

take a big inhale, and open to your right for your twisted half moon. Soften back through center, press your right fingertips to the ground, take a big inhale, and open to your left for your open half moon. Soften through your knees, step your top leg back, press down through your legs, and lift everything up, lifting your hips and arms up. Soften to warrior 2. Take a big inhale and lift up. Exhale and soften warrior 2. Tip back reverse. Tip up and over to your extended side angle, planting your forearm on your thigh and rolling your body open. Press down through your legs, take a big inhale, and lift up through warrior 2. Tip back reverse. Sweep through warrior 3, softening your knees and crawling your fingertips out in front of you. Let your back leg float up. Soften your knees and round up to stand hugging your left shin in with you for a squeeze. Roll around in your hips if that feels nice. Take a big inhale and lift up. Exhale and dive up and over your leg for your standing split. Relax your head and neck and roll around a bit in your hips to open up. When you're ready, soften your knees and step back to low lunge. Press down through your legs, take a big inhale, and lift up to high lunge. Exhale and soften back to low lunge. Make your way back to down dog, however feels great for you.

Repeat the phrase on the other side.

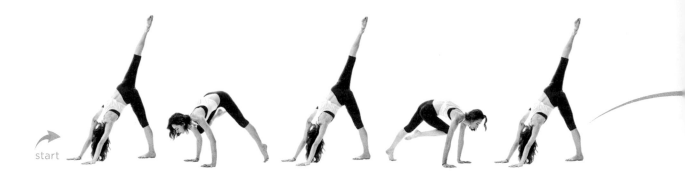

start

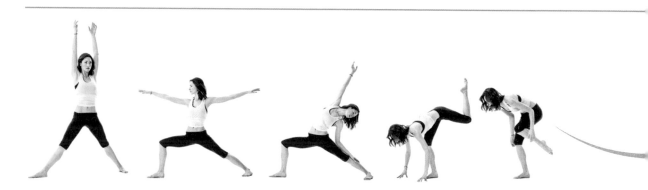

The first section here is nice to demonstrate mirroring in the front of the room. You can move to the side where people can see and hear you for the warrior 2 section and back up to the front for the balance movements. Handstand rocks is your moment to support a few people individually. Always keep an eye out for people who could use a little help. The more you get to know the people in the room, the more gracefully and easily you can position yourself to help.

Take a big inhale and lift your right leg up and back to down dog split. Arc your knee high and around to your right shoulder. Look forward; lean forward. When you're ready, lift your leg up and back to down dog split. Arc your knee down and across toward your left upper arm. Make a shelf. Look forward and lean forward. When you're ready, lift the leg up and back to down dog split. Step your foot on through to low lunge. Press down through your legs, take a big inhale, and lift up to high lunge. Exhale and twist to your left, letting your arms open wide. Inhale back to high lunge. Twice more like that. Exhale and twist toward your left and let your arms open wide. Inhale back up. One more time, exhale and twist toward your left, letting your arms open wide. Inhale back up and open to warrior 2. Spin your

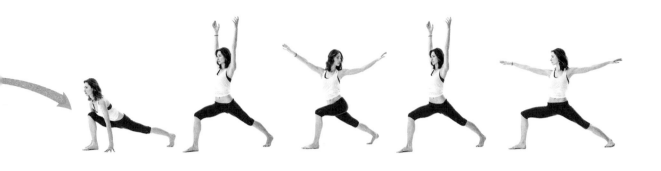

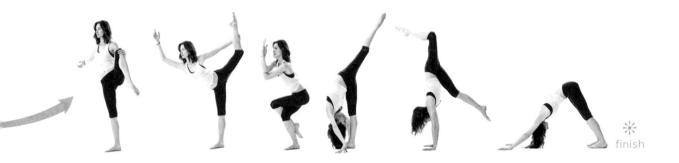

*finish

back heel to the ground, sink your hips, and settle your arms out to your sides. Soften here for a bit.

Take a big inhale and lift your hips and arms up. Exhale and soften back to warrior 2. Two more like that. Big inhale and fill up. Exhale and settle back. One more time, big inhale and open up. Exhale and soften to warrior 2. Tip back reverse warrior. Sweep it through to warrior 3, soften your knees, and crawl yourself forward, letting your back leg float on up. Soften your knees and round up to stand, bringing your left shin along with you for a squeeze. Roll around in your hips here to open up. Drop your knee toward the ground and catch hold of your foot with your left hand. Soften here for a moment. Take a big inhale and press your foot into your hand, opening your opposite arm up for your dancer. Soften here. Wrap your left leg up and over and your left arm under for your eagle. Sink through your hips and lift up through your fingertips. Unravel out of this and take a big inhale and lift up. Exhale, dive up and over your leg, plant your palms on the ground a bit in front of your front foot, and rock forward and back from your hips. If you'd rather roll around in your standing split, that's great too. Eventually we'll meet up in your down dog.

Repeat the phrase on the other side.

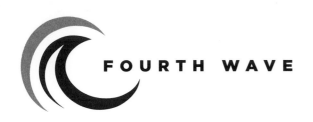

FOURTH WAVE

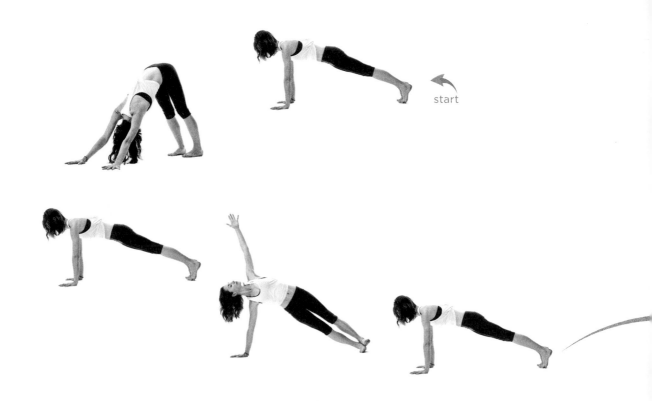

start

Use your voice and breath-body connection to demonstrate on your feet as you move through the group. You can put yourself on your feet where people can see and hear you on the side plank sides also.

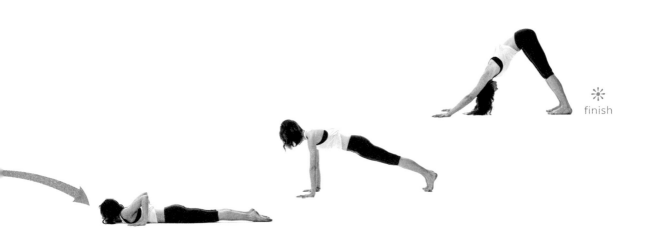

finish

Tuck your chin and round out to plank. Settle here for a moment. Sway a bit side to side or easy forward and back to open up a bit. When you're ready, lift your hips up and back to down dog. Tuck your chin and round back to plank. Shift your weight onto your right side, take a big inhale, and open your body to your left. When you're ready, come back to plank and open to your other side. When you're ready, come back to plank. Soften your elbows and lower to your belly. Press right back up. Twice more like that. Soften all the way down. Gently press back up. One more time, ease on down and all the way up and back to down dog. Settle here for a moment.

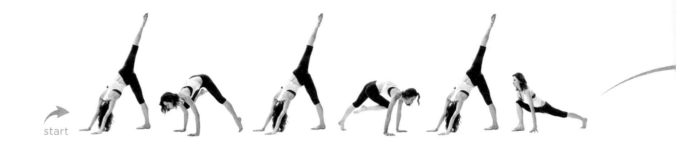

start

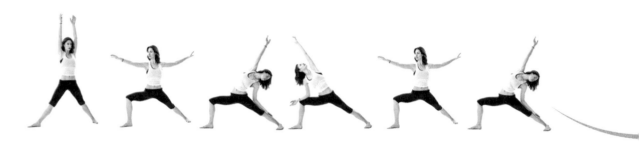

Knee hovers are great to support people with your voice and breath-body connection while you're on your feet in the mix of the group. Warrior 2 and reverse warrior are nice to demonstrate on the side of the room, facing people, where they can see and hear you.

When you're ready, take a big inhale and lift your right leg up and back to down dog split. Arc your knee high and around toward your right shoulder. Look forward and lean forward. When you're ready, bring your leg up and back to down dog split. Same thing across, arc your knee down and over toward your left upper arm. Make a shelf for the leg. Look forward and lean forward. When you're ready, take your leg up and back down to dog split. Step it on through to low lunge. Press down through your legs, take a big inhale, and lift up to high lunge. Exhale twist to your left, letting your arms open wide. Tip it back reverse. Tip forward, up, and over to your twisted half moon. Bring your right fingertips to the ground; soften through your knees as you twist around to your left. If you'd like to catch hold of your back foot as you twist around, go for that. If it doesn't feel nice, open back up. Take a big inhale and open here. Exhale soften through your middle and open up to your open half moon, right fingertips on the ground, opening to your left. If you'd like to catch hold of your foot behind you, go for that. If it doesn't feel nice, open back up. Soften through your knees, step your top foot back, press down

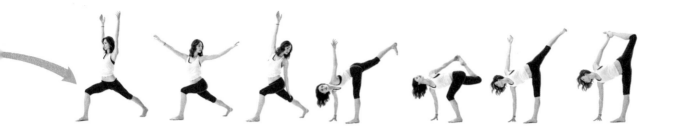

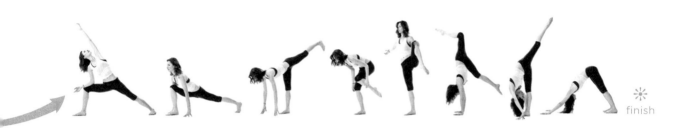

finish

through your legs, take a big inhale, and lift everything up, lifting your hips and arms up. Exhale soften to warrior 2. Tip back to reverse warrior. Tip up and over to your extended side angle, planting your forearm on your thigh and your opposite arm up and overhead. Roll your belly open if that feels nice. Press down through your legs, take a big inhale to lift up through your warrior 2, and tip back to reverse warrior. Tip up and over to your extended side angle. Roll open here.

When you're ready, come into a low lunge. Sink your hips and relax your head and neck.

Open your hips up a bit, soften your knees, and crawl yourself out to warrior 3. Soften your knees and round up to stand, hugging your shin along with you for a squeeze. Roll around a bit in the hips here if that feels nice. Take a big inhale and lift up. Exhale dive up and over, plant your palms on the ground a bit in front of your front foot, and rock forward and back a bit here. If you'd rather roll around in your standing split, that's great too. Eventually we'll meet in down dog.

Repeat the phrase on the other side.

FIFTH WAVE

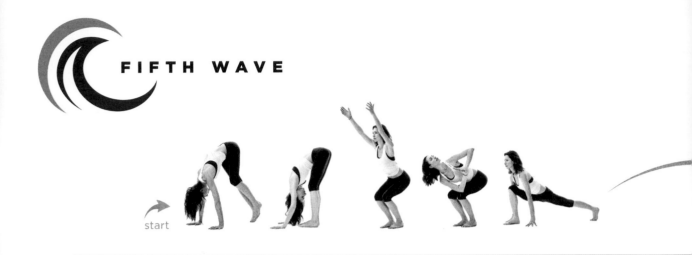

start

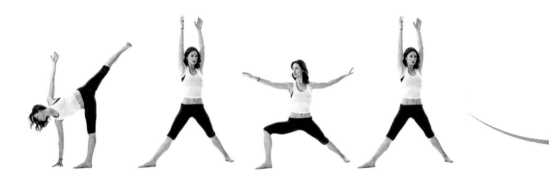

The first part of this phrase is nice to demonstrate facing and mirroring so people can see and follow you. You can come around to where people can see and hear you for warrior 2. Take time during warrior 2 to move around the room and check in with people, giving individual guidance to help people soften in the movement. For the balance movements, it's nice to make your way to the front of the room to demonstrate mirroring and facing. For the forearm section, make yourself ready to help and support people individually. Child's pose is another opportunity to make contact through touch and support.

When you're ready, walk your feet up to the top of your mat. Hands can walk too. Fold up and over your legs. Soften your knees and relax your head and neck. Sink through your hips, take a big inhale, and lift up into chair. Bring your palms together and twist toward your left. Shift your weight onto your right foot and step your left leg back to low lunge. Press down through your legs, take a big inhale, and lift up to high lunge. Exhale and twist toward your right, letting your arms open

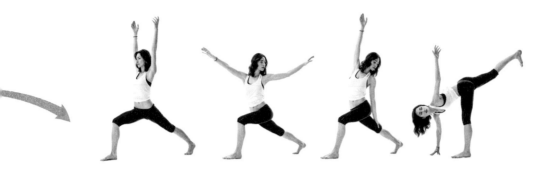

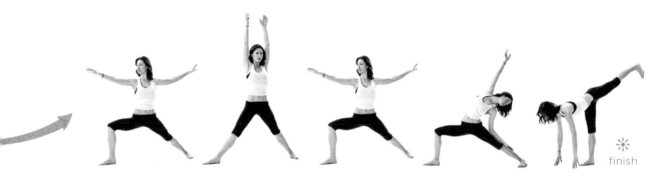

finish

wide. Tip back reverse. Tip up and over to your twisted half moon, bringing your left fingertips to the ground. Soften through your knees. Take a big inhale and open to your right. Soften through your middle, press your right fingertips to the ground, take a big inhale, and open to your left for your open half moon. Soften through your knees, step your top foot back, press down through your legs, take a big inhale, and lift everything up, lifting your hips and arms up. Exhale soften to warrior 2. We'll settle here for a few long, deep breaths. Let the inhale lift you up out of it and the exhale soften you a bit more, making this easier with each deep breath.

Take a big inhale and lift up and swivel around to warrior facing the back of the room. We'll settle here for a few long, deep breaths. If there is any tension hanging around, soften out of warrior, relax your head and neck, and rest. When you come back into warrior, let your inhales lift you up and your exhales soften even more.

Take a big inhale and lift up and swivel back around to your front for your warrior 2. Take a big inhale and lift up. Exhale soften back to warrior 2. Twice more like that, inhale and fill up. Exhale and settle back. One more time big inhale and open up. Exhale soften. Tip back to reverse warrior. Tip forward, sweeping through to your warrior 3, crawling your fingertips out and letting your back leg float up.

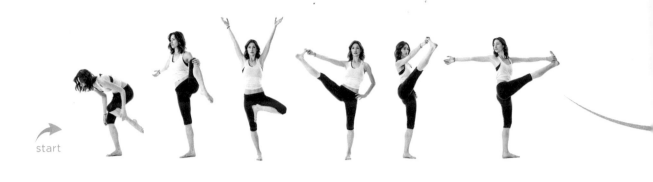

start

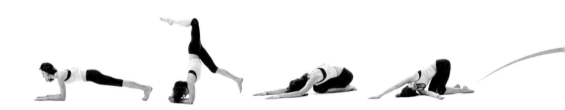

Soften your knees and round up to stand hugging your left shin in for a squeeze. Roll around a bit in your hips here to open up. We'll go for a few more balance movements. Your call. If you'd like to spend time in your tree, bring your foot into your thigh or on your ankle. If you'd like more to do, grab hold of your big toe or your heel with your first two fingers of your right hand. Soften here. Take a big inhale and extend your leg forward. Relax your head, neck, and shoulders. If you'd like to open the leg out to the side, go for that. When you're ready to bring it back forward, go for that. We'll turn it into a twist. Soften your knees and grab hold of the outside of your right foot with your left hand and twist to your right. Take a big inhale and open up here. Come back to center. Drop your knee down and catch hold of your foot behind you. Relax here. Take a big inhale and press your foot into your hand for dancer. Open your opposite arm up. Soften here and wrap your left leg up and around your right, left arm under your right for your eagle. Sink through your hips and lift up through your fingertips. When you're ready, unravel here. Take a big inhale and lift up. Exhale and dive up and over your leg, plant your palms on the ground a bit in front of your front foot and rock a bit forward and back. If you'd rather roll around in your standing split, that's great too. Eventually we'll meet in your low lunge.

Soften your knees; step your top leg back. Move your front foot out to the edge of your mat. Soften your back knee down to the ground and get into your hips a bit here. If you feel good here, stay here. If it feels better to soften your elbows and come down a bit more, go for that. Move softly and easily so you can find a nice place. If you feel good here, feel free to stay. If you'd like to spin around to your right side and

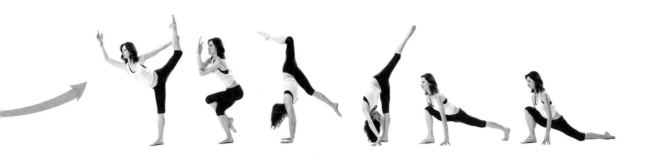

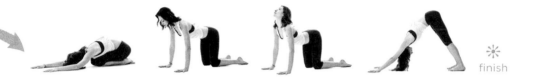

※
finish

catch hold of your back foot, go for that. If there is any pain or tweaking, ease on out. If you'd like to stay here and get into your hips, go for that. If you'd like to come into a forearm plank, come on down to your forearms; lean toward your left so much that you can slide your front foot behind you to your forearm plank. Stay here if you feel good. If you would like to walk your feet up toward your face, lifting your hips and belly, go for that. Take a big inhale and lift a leg up, lifting your hips and belly up. Exhale and soften back down. Roll through that a few times on each side. If you'd like a catch, I can catch you. If you'd like to rest in child's pose, that's great too. Eventually we'll meet up in child's pose. Rest here for a bit.

We'll open up the shoulders a bit. Staying in your child's pose, lift up your hips a bit and thread your right arm under your left, resting your right shoulder on the ground. Roll around a bit here to find a nice place to rest on your back. We'll hang here for a few breaths. When you're ready, come back to center and relax for a bit. When you're ready, lift your hips up a bit and thread your left arm under your right, resting your left shoulder on the ground. Roll around a bit here to find a nice place to rest. Breathe really fully and deeply. When you're ready, come back to your child's pose and relax.

Come back onto all fours when you're ready, and roll around a bit here to open up. Eventually we'll meet back in down dog. Take your time. When you feel good, tuck your toes, and let a big inhale do all the lifting for you. Soften back to down dog. Settle here for a bit.

Repeat the phrase on the other side.

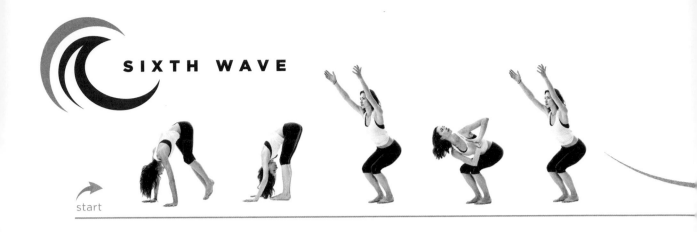

SIXTH WAVE

start

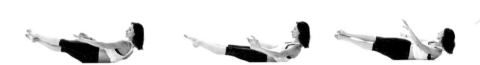

This is nice to demo mirroring and facing. You can also support people with your voice and breath-body connection while moving around the room. For crow it's nice to demonstrate how to do the movement and make your way to anyone who needs help. If you are pregnant and guiding, I would suggest not demonstrating boats or any movements that contract your belly or other movements that don't feel comfortable for you.

When you're ready, walk your feet up to the top of your mat. Hands can walk too. Fold up and over your legs. Soften your knees. Relax your head and neck. Sway a bit here if that feels nice. When you're ready, sink your hips, take a big inhale, and lift up to your chair. Bring your palms together and twist toward your left. Take a big inhale and lift up to your chair. Exhale and twist toward your right. Take a big inhale and come back to your chair. Exhale up and over your legs, interlacing your hands behind you for a nice shoulder release. Sway a bit here if that feels nice. When you're ready, relax your hands to the ground, put some weight into your arms, and sink your hips into a squat. Up to you if you'd like to relax your head and neck forward, or open up side to side to get into your hips or go for your crow. If you're going for your crow, try leaning back out of it, bringing your hands behind you. Relax here and see if you're movable. When you're ready, take a big inhale and bring your whole body forward. Look forward and lean forward. Exhale, soften back, and relax. Go through this a few times with your breath. When you're ready, we'll meet up on your hips, bringing your hands behind you to ease yourself down.

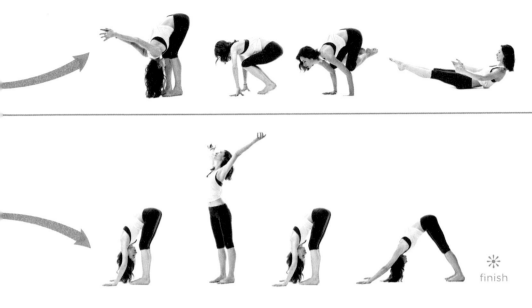

finish

Lift your shins up for your boat. Relax your shoulders. Lower halfway down, feet forward and head and shoulders back. Gently bring it right back up. Halfway down, and all the way up. Halfway down, and all the way up. A few more of these, halfway down, and all the way up. Halfway down, and all the way up. Ease on down, and all the way up. Ease on down, and all the way up. Three more times, ease on down, and all the way up. Halfway down, and bring it on up. Last one, ease on down, and all the way up.

Lower on your right side, bringing your right ribs to the ground, and all the way back up. Lower on your left side, and all the way up. A few more of these, lower to your right, and all the way up. And over to your left, and all the way up. Couple more times, over to your right, and all the way up, over to your left, and all the way up. One more time, over to your right, and all the way up, over to your left, and all the way up.

Bring it halfway down through the middle, and all the way up. A few more of these, lower halfway down, and all the way up. Easy in your shoulders, halfway down, and all the way up. Two more times, halfway down, and all the way up. One more, halfway down, and all the way up. Bring your feet to the ground, sit to the side, and bring your legs around behind you. Use the strength of your arms to lift yourself up into your standing forward bend. Relax your head and neck and soften here for a moment. When you're ready, round up to stand one notch at a time. Once you make it up, take a big inhale and float your arms out and up. Exhale and soften up and over your legs. We'll meet up in down dog in a bit. Roll through however feels great to unwind along the way.

SEVENTH WAVE

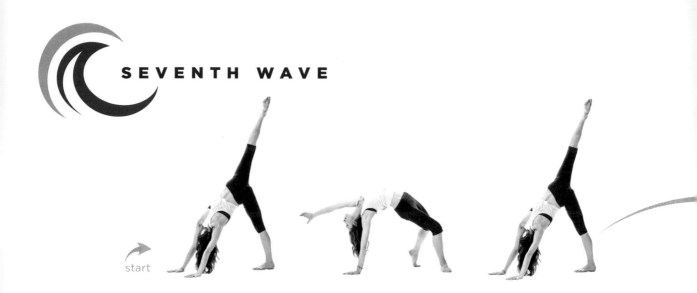

start

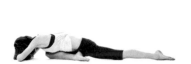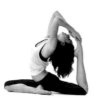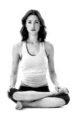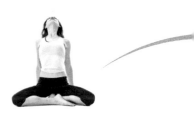

This is nice to demo on your feet, describing the movements with your voice and breath-body connection to help people with the directions and instructions. Pigeon and ankle to knee is your time to connect and support a few people individually.

When you're ready, take a big inhale and float your right leg up and back to down dog split. Open up so much that you tip over for your rock star. If you'd rather hang in your down dog split, that's great too. When you're ready, bring it back to your down dog split. Thread your foot down on the ground outside of your left hand. Float your right arm up, take a big inhale, and open up here for fallen triangle. When you're ready, bring it back to your down dog split. Soften your shin on through for your pigeon. Take a moment to get comfortable here. If there is any pain or tweaking in your knees, try bringing your foot closer to your body and sitting to the side on your hip. Take a big inhale and open up here. Either stay here or relax forward over your front shin. Take an easy stroll to one side or a nice gentle walk to the other side. Find a good place to relax for a bit.

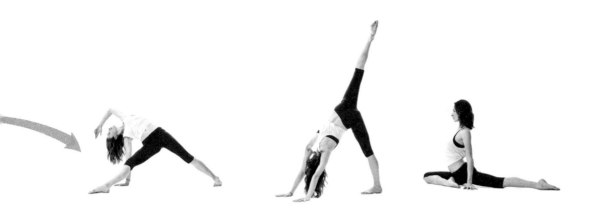

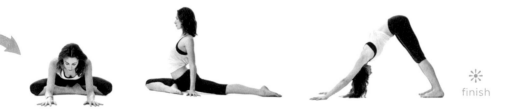

finish

If you feel good here, feel free to stay here. If you'd rather bring yourself up and take a nice twist to your right side, and an easy opening to your left side, go for that. If you'd like to lean forward, bend your back knee, and catch hold of your back foot, go for that. If there is any pain or tweaking, ease on out. When you're ready, unwind out of this one. Lean into your front hip and bring your back leg around. Stack your left leg on top of your right, bringing your left ankle on top of your right knee. If this doesn't feel good, bring your left leg on the ground in front of your right leg to sit easy. We'll breathe here for a bit. Bring your hands behind you on the ground, take a big inhale, and lean back. Either stay here, if this feels nice, or crawl yourself forward a bit to find a nice place to relax. Maybe crawl around to one side or the other to find a good spot, breathing fully and deeply. When you're ready, bring yourself back up and unwind back to your pigeon, leaning into your right hip and bringing your left leg around behind you. Eventually we'll meet in your down dog. Take your time if you'd like to spend a few more breaths in pigeon or roll through anything on the way back; move how it feels great for you to unwind.

Repeat the phrase on the other side.

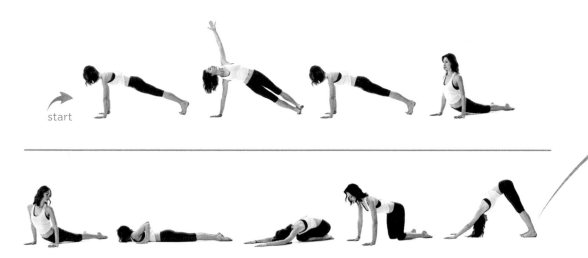

start

This is a nice place to support people with your voice and your breath-body connection while you're on your feet. You can be on the side, while on your feet, describing the movements where people can see you for the side planks, and connect through touch during child's pose and down dog.

Tuck your chin and round out to plank. Settle here for a moment. Lift your hips and shift onto your right side. Take a big inhale and open to your left. When you're ready, come back to center. Take a big inhale and open to your right. When you're ready, come back to center. Soften your knees and sink your hips, coming into your up dog. Sway a bit here if that feels nice. If this doesn't feel so great on your lower back, soften through your elbows and lower down a bit, getting into your middle and upper back. When you're ready, shift your hips back to child's pose. Relax here for a moment. When you're ready, come back onto all fours, spread your fingers wide, lift your hips, tuck your toes, and take a big inhale to lift up and back to down dog.

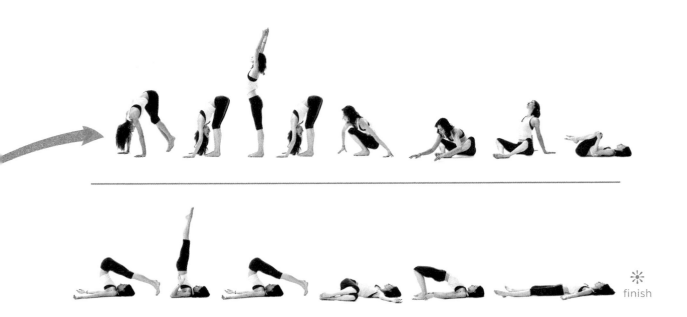

finish

When you're ready, walk on up to the top of your mat, one step at a time. Hands can walk too. Once you make it up, fold up and over your legs. Soften your knees and sway a bit if that feels nice. Round up to stand one notch at a time. Once you make it up, take a big inhale and float your arms out and up. Exhale and soften up and over your legs.

Soften your knees and press your palms on the ground; put some weight into your arms and come into a squat. Roll around a bit here to open up however it feels nice. When you're ready, bring your hands behind you and come to sit down easily. Do any forward bend that feels nice to you, bottoms of the feet together, legs apart, or legs forward. Take a big inhale and lean back and open up. Either stay here if this feels nice or guide yourself forward, exploring around to one side and the other, finding a nice place to breathe for a few moments. When you're ready, round on down to your back, carrying your knees along with you. Hug your knees into your chest and either rock side to side to open up, or round up and over for your plow. If plow doesn't feel nice on your back and neck, round gently down. If you'd like to evolve your plow into your shoulder stand, bring your palms to support your back and lift your legs up. Wherever you are, breathe really full and deep. Feel free to stay there as long as feels nice. When you're ready, ease on back down. Anything else you'd like to roll through before we rest. Maybe a gentle twist side to side or an easy bridge. Take your time. When you're ready, stretch out a bit. If there is any tension lingering around, take a big inhale through your nose and long exhale out through your mouth. Twice more just like that. When you're ready, rest here.

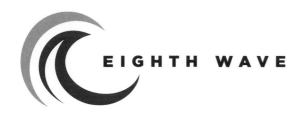

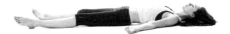

Here you have an opportunity to connect with several people through touch. There's nothing to guide with words here. Moving around the room, supporting people with touch, is great.

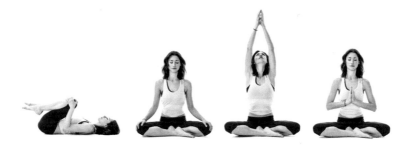

It's great to be in the front of the room sitting easily as you guide people to come out of the relaxation and meet them in easy seated for meditation.

Start to invite some more air back into your body. Roll around your wrists and ankles if that feels nice. Stretch out your arms overhead if that feels nice. When you're ready, hug your knees into your chest, and make your way up to sit in the easiest way.

Close your eyes and let your attention drift inward. Take a big inhale and float your arms up and overhead. Press your palms together and bring your thumbs to your heartbeat. Soften here for a moment. Take a big inhale through your nose. Exhale out through your mouth. Twice more like that, big inhale. Long exhale. One more time, big inhale, long exhale. Soften here for a moment.

Namaste and thank you for coming!

CLASS 5: Strala STRONG

THE PURPOSE

The purpose of STRONG is to build strength and mobility evenly and work on staying calm, focused, and soft during simple and challenging moments alike.

THE DESCRIPTION

Strala STRONG is a moving flow that builds strength, balance, and flexibility evenly in the body. Calm ease is carried through simple and challenging movements alike. You get happy and healthy from the inside out.

FIRST WAVE

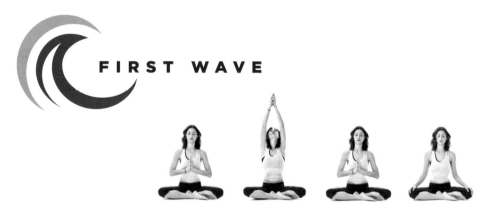

Begin sitting in the front of the room, facing the group. Demonstrate along with the group here.

Sit easy, however you can be comfortable. Close your eyes and let your attention rest a bit deeper inward. Take a big inhale and float your arms up and overhead. Press your palms together and bring your thumbs to your heartbeat. Soften here for a moment. All together take a big inhale through your nose. Long exhale out through your mouth. Twice more like that. Big inhale. Long exhale. One more time, big inhale. Long exhale. When you're ready, relax your hands on your thighs.

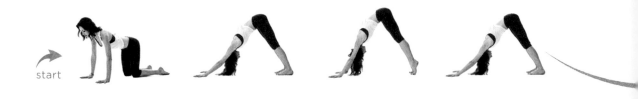

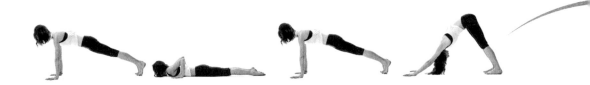

Coming onto all fours and heading into down dog is a nice thing to show for knee safety reasons. Sit to the side and bring your legs around, instead of bringing your torso through your legs in a crossed position. Even if this move is easy for you, it's stressful on the knees. If people do what you do, which is what is mostly the case, they'll injure their knees. Always show the process of the movement over any destination of a pose.

Down dog is a nice place to make physical contact with people. Since you have a movement repeated here three times, you have an opportunity to make contact with three people. Being easy in the room and relaxed in your body will help you navigate to make contact. Forward bend is another nice place to make contact.

When you're ready, sit to the side and come around and onto all fours. Spread your fingers wide, tuck your toes, take a big inhale, and lift your hips up and back to down dog. Soften here for a moment. Press into one heel and then the other if that feels nice to open up a bit. Take a big inhale and lift up on to your tiptoes. Exhale, soften, and relax. Twice more like that, big inhale lift up. Exhale, soften, and

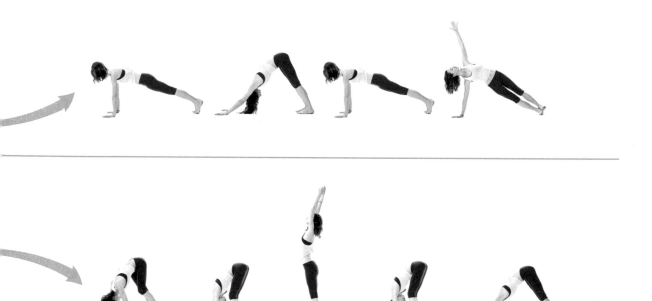

※ finish

relax. One more time, big inhale and lift. Exhale and soften back down. Tuck your chin and round out to plank. Settle here for a moment. Sway side to side or easy forward and back to open up a bit. When you're ready, lift your hips up and back to down dog. Tuck your chin and round back to plank. Shift your weight onto your right hand and the outside edge of your right foot and open your body to your left. Hold here for a few seconds. Come back to plank and move to the other side.

When you're ready, come back to center. Soften your elbows and lower to your belly. Press right back up. Twice more like that. Soften all the way down. Gently press back up. One more time, ease on down and all the way up and back to down dog. Settle here for a moment.

When you're ready, walk on up to the front of your mat. Hands can walk too. Once you make it up, fold up and over your legs. Relax your head and neck. Sway a bit here if that feels nice. When you're ready, round up to stand one notch at a time. When you make it up, float your arms up and out. Easy exhale and soften back over your legs. Plant your palms and make your way back to down dog, either stepping back or rolling through whatever feels great.

SECOND WAVE

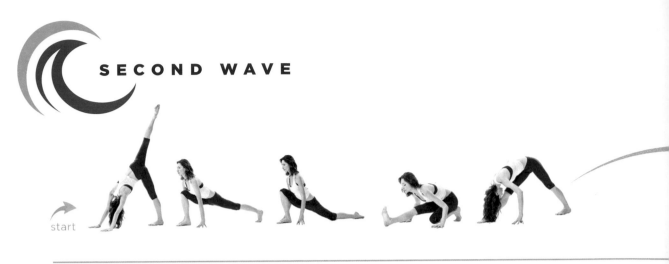

start

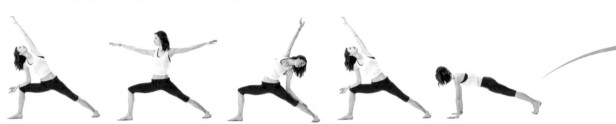

After down dog split, this phrase is nice to demonstrate from the front, mirroring and facing the group. You could also guide this phrase while working your way through the group, moving around gracefully, positioning yourself where people can see and hear you, and using your voice and breath-body connection.

Take a big inhale and lift your right leg up and back to down dog split. Open your hips and shoulders if that feels nice. Step your foot on through to low lunge. Soften here for a moment. When you're ready, ease your back knee down. If it feels nice to bring your torso low inside your font leg, go for that. If it feels nice to stay a bit higher and open up, that's great too. Breathe fully and deeply. When you're ready, bring your fingertips to the ground on either side of your front foot, tuck your back toes, and sink your hips toward your back heel for your runner's stretch. Relax your torso over your front leg. Sway a bit here if that feels nice. When you're ready, crawl yourself back to your low lunge, press your fingertips on the ground, and lift your hips up. Relax your torso over your front leg. Sway a bit here if that feels nice.

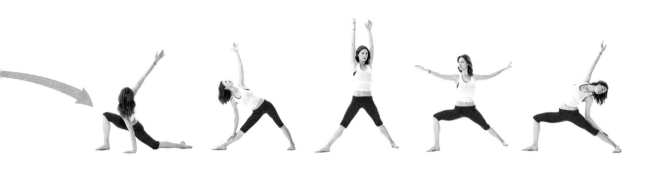

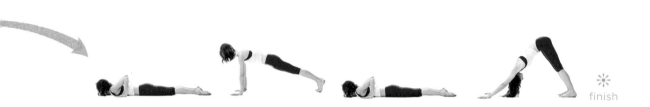

finish

Soften through your knees, press your left fingertips on the ground, take a big inhale, and open up to your right, floating your right arm up. We'll trade sides. Soften through your knees, press your right fingertips on the ground, spin your back heel down, take a big inhale, and open to your triangle. Soften through your knees, press down through your legs, take a big inhale, and lift up, lifting your hips and arms up overhead. Soften to warrior 2. Take a big inhale and lift up, lifting your hips and arms up. Settle back to warrior 2. One more time, big inhale and lift up. Exhale and soften back warrior 2. Tip back to reverse warrior. Tip up and over extended side angle, press your right forearm on your thigh, and open your opposite arm overhead. Roll your torso open. Press down through your legs, take a big inhale, and lift back through warrior 2, tip back reverse. Tip up and over to your extended side angle. Rolling open here. When you're ready, bring your palms down to the ground on either side of your front foot and step back to plank. Soften down to your belly. Press right back up. Twice more like that, ease on down, and press right back up. Last time, soften on down and press right back up and back to down dog.

Repeat the phrase on the other side.

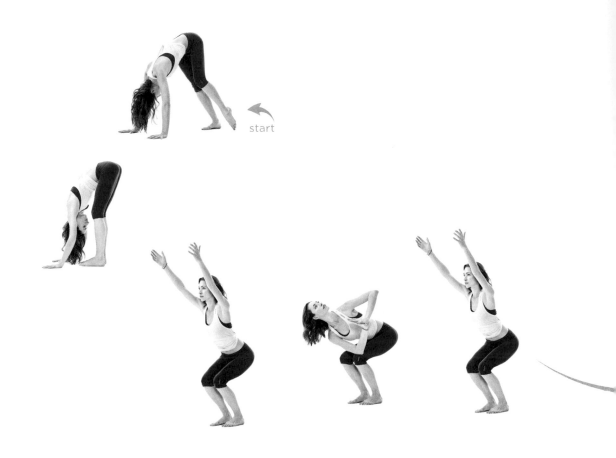

start

Crow is great to demo either in the front of the room or alongside anyone who is having trouble relaxing through the movement. To help individuals, come alongside them and show them with your demonstration how they can easily rock forward and back with their breath. Usually what happens is they are jumping or stopping their movement in the pose, which stops the ability for the movement to happen effectively. Often it's as simple as showing them they can look more forward, and that is the key for them to be able to accomplish this move with ease. Make sure to show the *process* in your own body, much more than any finished position.

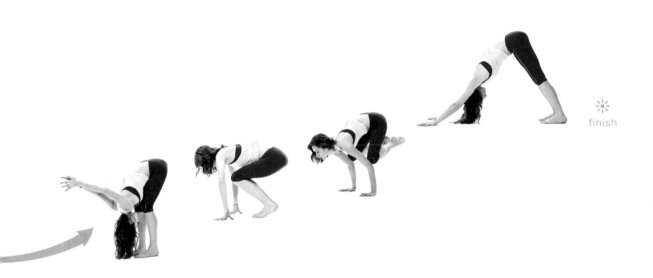

finish

When you're ready, take a walk up to the top of your mat. Hands can walk too. Once you get there, fold up and over your legs. Soften your knees a bit here and relax your head and neck. When you're ready, sink your hips, take a big inhale, and lift up to your chair. Bring your palms together and twist toward your left. Take a big inhale back to your chair. Exhale and twist toward your right. Big inhale back to your chair. Exhale, fold up and over your legs, and interlace your hands behind you for a shoulder release. Soften your knees and sway a bit here if that feels nice. Relax your head and neck. When you're ready, bring your hands to the ground in front of you. Bring some weight into your arms and sink your hips to your squat. Sway a bit here to open up your hips and belly if that feels nice. Up to you, either stay with this or, if you want to go for your crow, plant your palms on the ground in front of you, take a big inhale, lean forward, and look forward. Exhale, soften back, and relax. Go for this a few times with your breath. As you inhale squeeze your knees around your arms, looking forward and leaning forward. Exhale, soften back, and relax. Roll through this a few times with your breath, and when you're ready, make your way back to down dog however feels great for you.

THIRD WAVE

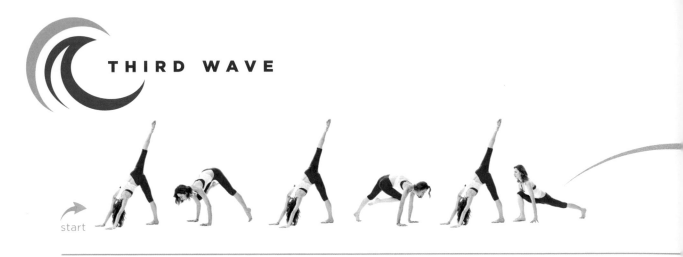

start

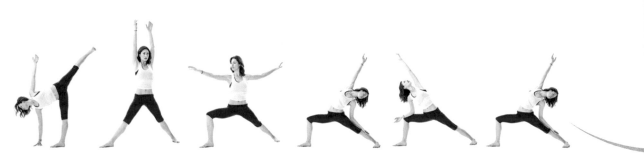

This is nice to demo from the front of the room so people can see and mirror your movements. All except your knee hovers and crosses. During these moves, make your way through the group, supporting people with your voice and breath-body connection.

Take a big inhale and lift your right leg up and back to down dog split. Arc your knee high and around toward your right shoulder. Lean forward. Look forward. Moving from your hips. When you're ready, lift the leg back to down dog split. Arc your knee down and across your body toward your left upper arm. Make a shelf for the leg with your arms. Lean forward. Look forward. When you're ready, lift the leg up and back to down dog split. Step your foot on through to low lunge. Take a big inhale and lift up to high lunge. Bring your palms together, thumbs to your heartbeat. Take a big inhale and lift up. Exhale and twist toward your left, bringing your right elbow outside your thigh. Up to you, either stay here or open up your arms, bringing your left fingertips to the ground, right arm opening upward, staying soft. When you're ready, bring both fingertips to the ground on either side of your front foot, lift your hips up, and relax your torso over your front leg. Sway a bit here if that feels nice. Soften your knees, crawl your fingertips out in front of you, and let

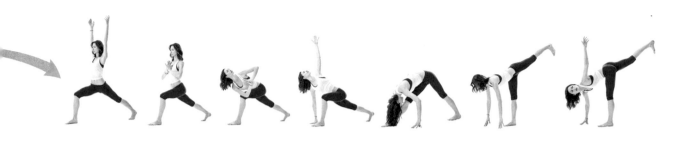

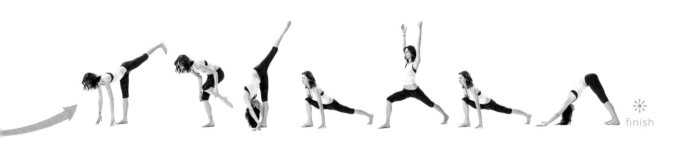

finish

your back leg float up into warrior 3. Soften your knees, press your right fingertips on the ground, take a big inhale, and open your body to your left for your twisted half moon. Soften through your center, take a big inhale, and open to your left for your open half moon. Soften through your knees, and reach your arms forward as your reach your back leg back. Press down through your legs, take a big inhale, and lift your hips and arms up. Soften into your warrior 2. Tip back reverse warrior. Tip up and over to your extended angle, pressing your forearm on your thigh and your opposite arm up and overhead. Give yourself a chance to roll open here. When you're ready, take a big inhale and lift up and back to reverse warrior. Sweep through to your warrior 3, crawling your fingertips out in front of you and letting your back leg float up. Soften your knees and round up to stand, hugging your left shin in toward your chest for a squeeze. Roll around in the hips here if that feels nice. Take a big inhale to lift up. Exhale and dive up and over your leg for your standing split. Drop your head and neck, planting your palms on the ground a bit in front of your front foot. Roll around a bit in your hips here to open up. When you're ready, soften your knees and step back to your low lunge. Take a big inhale and lift up to your high lunge. Exhale back through your low lunge and make your way to down dog however feels great for you.

Repeat the phrase on the other side.

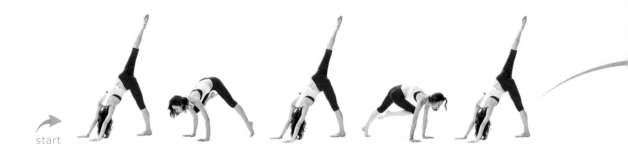

start

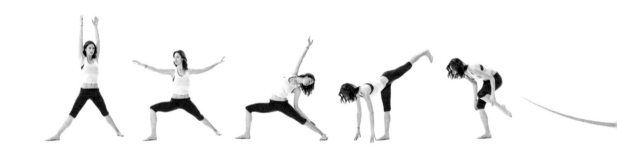

The beginning of this phrase is good to support with your voice and breath-body connection while you're moving through the room. Starting with low lunge, it's nice to demo mirroring and facing the group.

Take a big inhale and lift your right leg up and back to down dog split. Arc your knee high and around toward your right shoulder. Lean forward. Look forward. Moving from your hips. When you're ready, lift the leg back to down dog split. Arc your knee down and across your body toward your left upper arm. Make a shelf for the leg with your arms. Lean forward. Look forward. When you're ready, lift the leg up and back to down dog split. Step your foot on through to low lunge. Take a big inhale and lift up to high lunge. Exhale and twist to your left, letting your arms open wide. Tip back and reverse. Tip up and over to your twisted half moon, bringing your left fingertips to the ground and opening your body to your right. Soften as you spin around. Soften through your center, take a big inhale, and open to your left for your open half moon. Soften through your knees, reach your arms forward as your reach your back leg back. Press down through your legs, take a big inhale, and lift your hips and arms up. Soften into your warrior 2. Tip back reverse warrior.

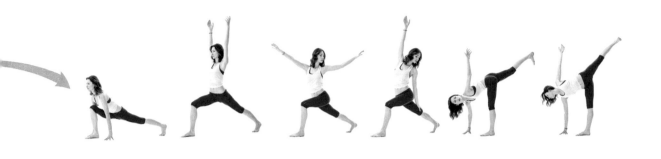

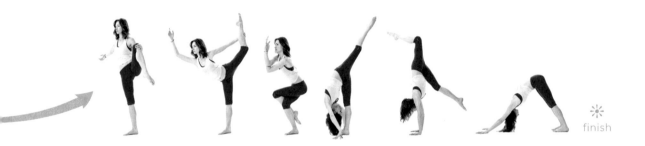

finish

Sweep through to your warrior 3, crawling your fingertips out in front of you and letting your back leg float up. Soften your knees and round up to stand, hugging your left shin in toward your chest for a squeeze. Roll around in the hips here if that feels nice. Drop your knee toward the ground and catch hold of your foot with your left hand. Soften here. Take a big inhale and lift up into your dancer, pressing your foot into your hand and opening your opposite arm up. When you're ready, soften here, wrap your left leg up and around your right, left arm under your right for your eagle. Sink through your hips and lift up through your fingertips. When you're ready, unravel. Take a big inhale to lift up. Exhale and dive up and over your leg toward your standing split. Plant your palms on the ground a bit in front of your front foot. If you'd like to rock forward and back, go for that. If you'd rather roll around in your standing split for a few breaths, that's great too. Eventually we'll meet in up in down dog. If you're rocking, take a big inhale and rock forward, easy exhale and soften back. Keep your knees soft and move your whole body from your hips. When you're ready, we'll meet up in down dog.

Repeat the phrase on the other side.

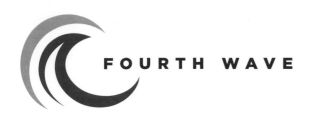

FOURTH WAVE

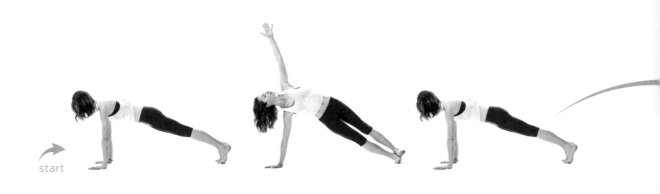

start

For the planks, it is nice to be on the side where people can see you on your feet. When you are guiding them to the second side, you have an opportunity to move and position yourself to the other side of the room and open up with everyone also.

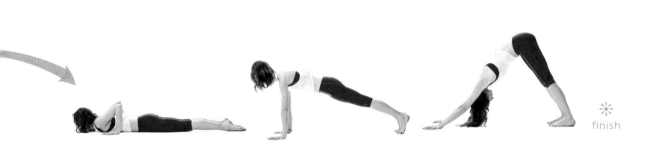

*
finish

Tuck your chin and round out to plank. Lift up your hips and roll onto your right side. Take a big inhale and open to your left. When you're ready, come back to center, take a big inhale, and open to your right. When you're ready, come back to plank. Soften your elbows and lower to your belly. Gently press right back up. Twice more like that, soften down. And gently press right back up. One more time, ease on down, and this time press right up and back to down dog.

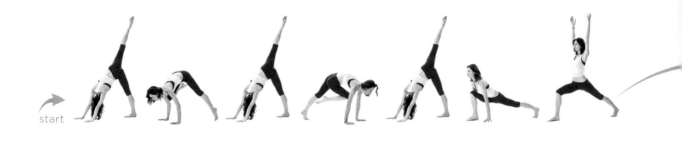

start

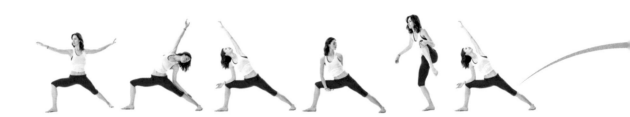

This is nice to demonstrate mirroring and facing or you could also support people with your voice and breath-body connection while moving around the room. Handstand rocks is your time to help a few people individually.

When you're ready, take a big inhale and lift your right leg up and back to down dog split. Arc your knee high and around toward your right shoulder. Look forward and lean forward. When you're ready, bring your leg up and back to down dog split. Same thing across, arc your knee down and over toward your left upper arm. Make a shelf for the leg. Look forward and lean forward. When you're ready, take your leg up and back to down dog split. Step it on through to low lunge. Press down through your legs, take a big inhale, and lift up to high lunge. Exhale, twist to your left, and let your arms open wide. Tip it back reverse. Tip forward, up, and over to your twisted half moon. Bring your left fingertips to the ground, and soften through your knees as you twist around to your right. If you'd like to catch hold of your back foot as you twist around, go for that. If it doesn't feel nice, open back up. Take a big inhale and open here. Exhale, soften through your middle, and open up to your open half moon, right fingertips on the ground opening to your left. If you'd like to catch hold of your foot behind you, go for that. If it doesn't feel nice, open back up. Soften through your knees, step your top foot back, press down through your legs, take a big inhale, and

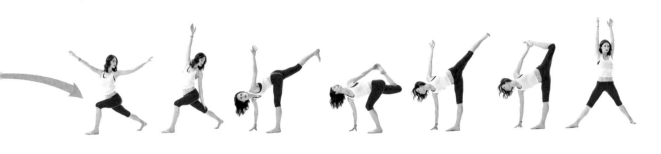

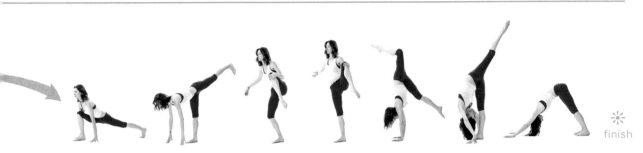

*
finish

lift everything up, lifting your hips and arms up. Exhale soften to warrior 2. Tip back to reverse warrior. Tip up and over to your extended side angle, planting your forearm on your thigh and your opposite arm up and overhead. Roll your belly open if that feels nice. Up to you, stay here if this feels nice, or if you'd like to play with a wrap, drop your top arm around your back and your bottom arm under your thigh, hooking fingers if that's easy. If you can't breathe here or if it doesn't feel great, come out of it a bit. Lift your hips, look forward, lean forward, and bring your back foot through to meet your front. Press down through your left leg and come up to stand. If the wrap is happening, open the leg if that feels nice. If it feels better to hug the shin and roll around in your hips, that's great too. When you're ready, we'll retrace back to extended side angle, opening up in a half moon on the way back if you'd like. Once you make it back down, press down through your legs and roll your torso open. When you're ready, come into a low lunge. Sink your hips and relax your head and neck.

Lift your hips and crawl yourself out to warrior 3. Soften your knees and round up to stand, hugging your shin along with you for a squeeze. Roll around a bit in the hips here if that feels nice. Take a big inhale and lift up. Exhale, dive up and over, and plant your palms on the ground a bit in front of your front foot and rock forward and back a bit here. If you'd rather roll around in your standing split, that's great too. Eventually we'll meet in down dog.

Repeat the phrase on the other side.

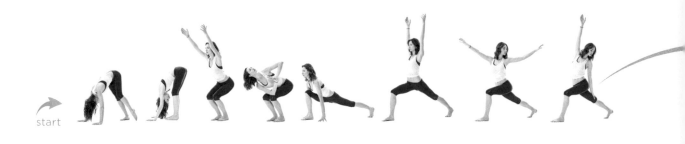

start

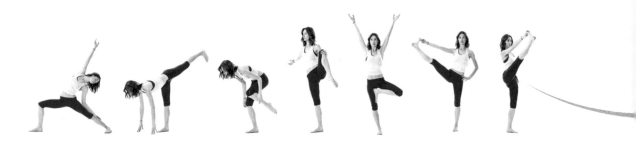

This phrase is nice to demo mirroring and facing the group, or making your way to the side where people are facing to demonstrate there. When the warrior 2 hold comes around, this is a nice place to go around and help anyone having a tough time or holding extra tension. Usually poor body position can be easily remedied by mirroring someone and showing a good position they can be in for warrior 2. When it is handstand exploration time, make sure to go and get involved in helping people individually.

When you're ready, walk your feet up to the top of your mat. Hands can walk too. Fold up and over your legs. Soften your knees and relax your head and neck. Sink through your hips, take a big inhale, and lift up into chair. Bring your palms together and twist toward your left. Shift your weight onto your right foot and step your left leg back to low lunge. Press down through your legs, take a big inhale, and lift up to high lunge. Exhale and twist toward your left, let your arms open wide. Tip back reverse. Tip up and over to your twisted half moon, bringing your left fingertips to the ground. Soften through your knees. Take a big inhale and open to your right. Soften through your middle, press your right fingertips to the ground, take a big inhale, and open to your left for your open half moon. Soften through your knees, step your top foot back, press down through your legs, take a big inhale, and lift everything up, lifting your hips and arms up. Exhale soften to warrior 2. We'll hang here for a bit. If there is any tension lingering, drop your arms, soften your knees, and roll around a bit from your middle. When you're ready, come back into your warrior 2. Let your inhales lift you up a bit and your exhales soften, making this easier with every big, deep breath. We'll stay here for several long, deep breaths.

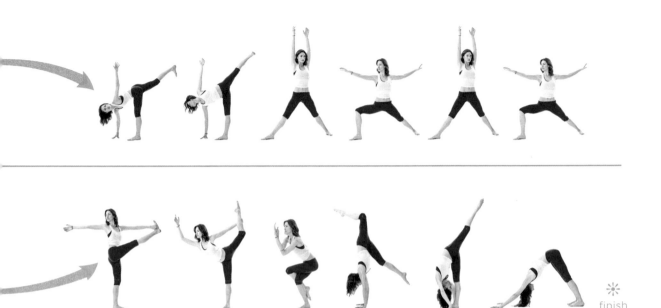

finish

Take a big inhale and lift up, lifting your hips and arms up. Exhale and settle back to warrior 2. Twice more like that, big inhale and lift. Easy exhale and soften. One more time, big inhale and fill up. Exhale and relax back to warrior 2. Tip back to reverse warrior. Sweep through to your warrior 3, soften your knees, crawl your fingertips forward, and let your back leg float up. Soften your knees and round up to stand, hugging your left shin in for a squeeze. Roll around a bit in your hips here to open up. We'll go for a few more balance movements. Your call. If you'd like to spend time in your tree, bring your foot into your thigh or on your ankle. If you'd like more to do, grab hold of your big toe with your first two fingers of your right hand, or grab your heel. Soften here. Take a big inhale and extend your leg forward. Relax your head, neck, and shoulders. If you'd like to open the leg out to the side, go for that. When you're ready to bring it back forward, go for that. We'll turn it into a twist. Soften your knees and grab hold of the outside of your right foot with your left hand and twist to your right. Take a big inhale and open up here. Come back to center. Drop your knee down and catch hold of your foot behind you. Relax here. Take a big inhale and press your foot into your hand for dancer. Open your opposite arm up. Soften here and wrap your left leg up and around your right, left arm under your right for your eagle. Sink through your hips and lift up through your fingertips. When you're ready, unravel here. Take a big inhale and lift up. Exhale and dive up and over your leg, plant your palms on the ground a bit in front of your front foot, and rock a bit forward and back. If you'd rather roll around in your standing split, that's great too. Eventually we'll meet in your down dog.

Repeat the phrase on the other side.

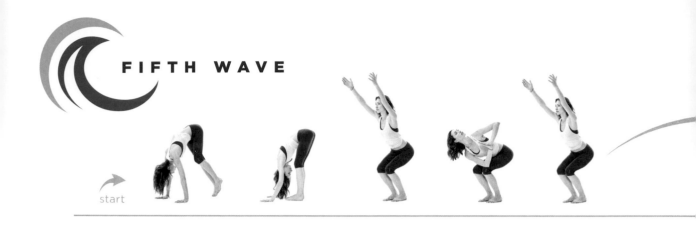

FIFTH WAVE

start

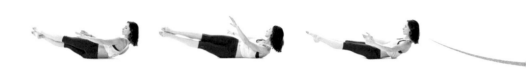

This is nice to demo mirroring and facing. You can also support people with your voice and breath-body connection while moving around the room. For crow, it's nice to demonstrate the movements and then take the time while people are exploring to go and help anyone that seems to want help. If you are pregnant and guiding, I would suggest not demonstrating boats or any movements that contract your belly or other movements that don't feel comfortable for you.

When you're ready, walk your feet up to the top of your mat. Hands can walk too. Fold up and over your legs. Soften your knees. Relax your head and neck. Sway a bit here if that feels nice. When you're ready, sink your hips, take a big inhale, and lift up to your chair. Bring your palms together and twist toward your left. Take a big inhale and lift up to your chair. Exhale and twist toward your left. Take a big inhale and come back to your chair. Exhale up and over your legs, interlacing your hands behind you for a nice shoulder release. Sway a bit here if that feels nice. When you're ready, relax your hands to the ground, put some weight into your arms, and sink your hips into a squat. Up to you if you'd like to relax your head and neck forward, or open up side to side to get into your hips or go for your crow here. If you're going for your crow, try starting by leaning back out of it, bringing your hands behind you. Relax here and see if you're movable. When you're ready, take a big inhale and bring your whole body forward. Look forward and lean forward. Exhale, soften back, and

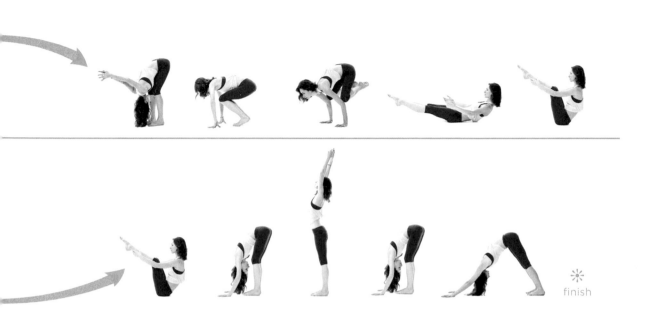

relax. Go through this a few times with your breath. When you're ready, we'll meet up on your hips, bringing your hands behind you to ease yourself down.

Lift your shins up for your boat. Relax your shoulders. Lower halfway down, feet forward and head and shoulders back. Gently bring it right back up. Halfway down, and all the way up. Halfway down, and all the way up. A few more of these, halfway down, and all the way up. Halfway down, and all the way up. Ease on down, and all the way up. Ease on down, and all the way up. Three more times, ease on down, and all the way up. Halfway down, and bring it on up. Last one, ease on down, and all the way up.

Lower on your right side, bringing your right ribs to the ground, and all the way back up. Lower on your left side, and all the way up. A few more of these, lower to your right, and all the way up. And over to your left, and all the way up. Couple more times, over to your right, and all the way up, over to your left, and all the way up. One more time, over to your right, and all the way up, over to your left, and all the way up.

Bring it halfway down through the middle, and all the way up. A few more of these, lower halfway down, and all the way up. Easy in your shoulders, halfway down, and all the way up. Two more times, halfway down, and all the way up. One more halfway down and all the way up. Bring your feet to the ground, sit to the side, and bring your legs around behind you. Use the strength of your arms to lift yourself up into your standing forward bend. Relax your head and neck and soften here for a moment. When you're ready, round up to stand one notch at a time. Once you make it up, take a big inhale and float your arms out and up. Exhale and soften up and over your legs. We'll meet up in down dog in a bit. Roll through whatever feels great to unwind along the way.

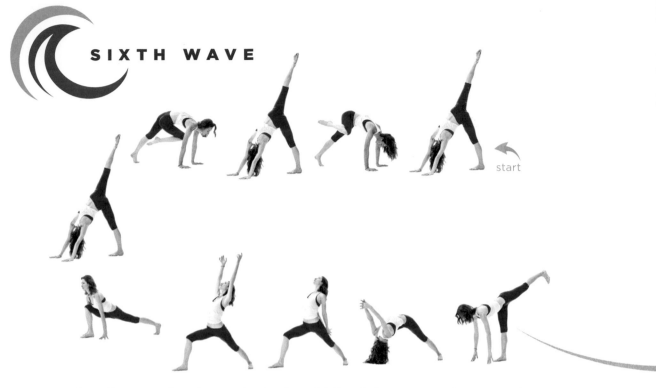

SIXTH WAVE

start

Hip rolls are a nice time to be in the middle of the group, where people can see you behind them when they are in down dog and going through the down dog split movements. You can show the movements while walking through the room by moving from your middle and letting the movement come through your arms. For warrior 1 it's nice to make your way to the front to demo and mirror. Forearm rocks are an opportunity to help people individually or support people in child's pose.

Take a big inhale and lift your right leg up and back to down dog split. Arc your knee high and around to your right shoulder, bring it across your body toward your left shoulder, and open it back up and back to down dog split. Bring your knee down and across your body toward your left shoulder, open it up, and sweep it back to down dog split. One more round like that. Arc your knee high and around right, across to your left, open it up and back to down dog split. Now down and around to your left, open it up and all the way back to down dog split. Step it on through to low lunge, ground your back heel down, press down through your legs, take a big inhale, and lift up to your warrior 1. Soften here for a moment. Soften your knees and roll around your hips here to find a good place. Breathe here for a moment.

When you're ready, drop your hands behind you, interlace them, take a big inhale, and open up. Exhale and fold up and over your legs. Twice more like that. Press down through your legs, take a big inhale, and open back up. Exhale and fold up and over your legs. Press down through your legs, take a big inhale, and open

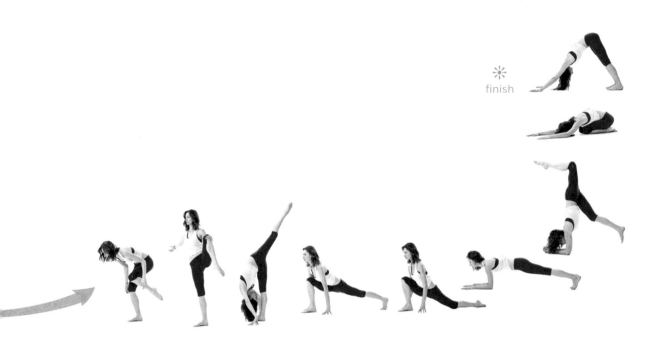

❄ finish

back up. Lean back, come onto your back toes, and bring yourself forward into your warrior 3. Soften your knees and round up to stand, bringing your left shin along with you for a squeeze. Roll around in your hips here if that feels nice. Take a big inhale and open up. Exhale and dive up and over for your standing split. Plant your palms on the ground a bit in front of your front foot. Roll around a bit in your hips here to take some of the weight out of your legs. When you're ready, we'll meet up in a low lunge. Soften your knees; step your top leg back. Move your front foot out to the edge of your mat. Soften your back knee down to the ground and get into your hips a bit here. Up to you—if you feel good here, stay here. If you feel better to soften your elbows and come down a bit more, go for that. Move softly and easily so you can find a nice place. If you feel good here, feel free to stay here. If you'd like to spin around to your right side, catch hold of your back foot, go for that. If there is any pain or tweaking, ease on out. If you'd like to stay here and get into your hips, go for that. If you'd like to come into a forearm plank, come on down to your forearms, and lean toward your left so much that you can slide your front foot behind you to your forearm plank. Stay here if you feel good. If you would like to walk your feet up toward your face, lifting your hips and belly, go for that. Take a big inhale and lift a leg up, lifting your hips and belly up. Exhale and soften back down. Roll through that a few times on each side. If you'd like a catch, I can catch you. If you'd like to rest in child's pose, that's great too. Eventually we'll meet up in down dog. Take your time.

Repeat the phrase on the other side.

SEVENTH WAVE

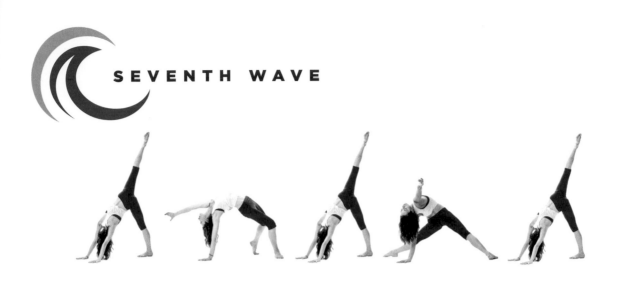

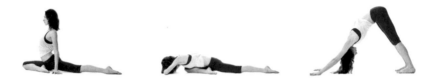

This is a nice time to support people with your voice and breath-body connection as you're on your feet. Pigeon is your time to connect and support a few people individually.

When you're ready, take a big inhale and float your right leg up and back to down dog split. Open up so much that you tip over for your rock star. If you'd rather hang in your down dog split, that's great too. When you're ready, bring it back to your down dog split. Thread your foot down on the ground outside of your left hand. Float your right arm up, take a big inhale, and open up here. When you're ready, bring it back to your down dog split. Soften your shin on through for your pigeon. Take a moment to get comfortable here. If there is any pain or tweaking in your knees, try bringing your foot closer to your body and sitting to the side on your hip. Take a big inhale and open up here. Either stay here or relax forward over your front shin. Take an easy stroll to one side or a nice gentle walk to the other side. Find a good place to relax for a bit.

If you feel good here, feel free to stay here. If you'd rather bring yourself up and take a nice twist to your right side, and an easy opening to your left side, go for that. If you'd like to lean forward, bend your back knee, and catch hold of your back foot, go for that. If there is any pain or tweaking, ease on out. Eventually we'll meet in your down dog. Take your time if you'd like to spend a few more breaths in pigeon or roll through anything on the way back; move how it feels great for you to unwind.

Repeat the phrase on the other side.

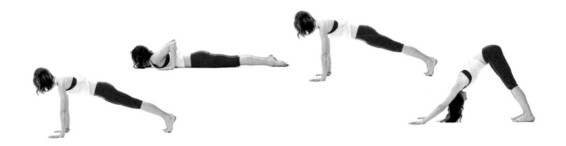

This is a nice time to support people with your voice and breath-body connection as you're on your feet.

Tuck your chin and round out to plank. Settle here for a bit. Ease on down to your belly. Gently press right back up. Twice more like that. Ease on down and right back up. One more time, ease on down and right up and back to down dog.

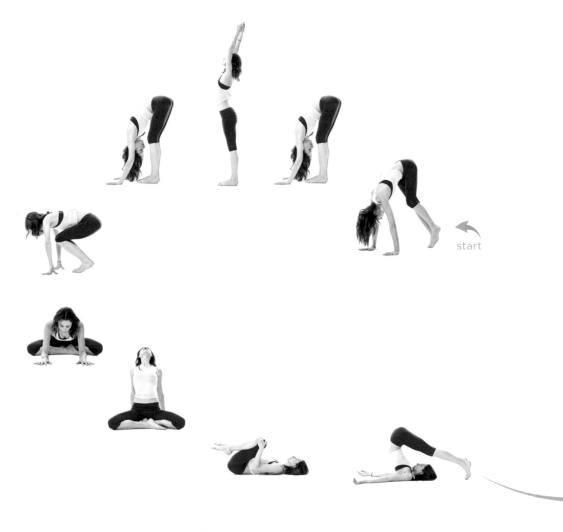

start

When you're ready, walk on up to the top of your mat, one step at a time. Hands can walk too. Once you make it up, fold up and over your legs. Soften your knees and sway a bit if that feels nice. Round up to stand one notch at a time. Once you make it up, take a big inhale and float your arms out and up. Exhale and soften up and over your legs.

Soften your knees and press your palms on the ground, put some weight into your arms, and come into a squat. Roll around a bit here to open up how it feels nice. When you're ready, bring your hands behind you and come to sit down easily. Any forward bend that feels nice to you, bottoms of your feet together, legs apart, or legs forward. Take a big inhale and lean back and open up. Either stay here if this feels nice or guide yourself forward, exploring around to one side and the

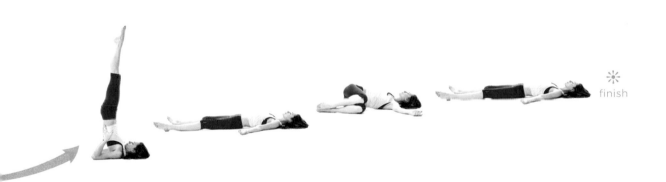

finish

other, finding a nice place to breathe for a few moments. When you're ready, round on down to your back, carrying your knees along with you. Hug your knees into your chest and either rock side to side to open up, or round up and over for your plow. If plow doesn't feel nice on your back and neck, round gently down. If you'd like to evolve your plow into your shoulder stand, bring your palms to support your back and lift your legs up. Wherever you are, breathe really fully and deeply. Feel free to stay there as long as feels nice. When you are ready, ease on back down. Anything else you'd like to roll through before we rest. Maybe a gentle twist side to side. Take your time. When you're ready, stretch out a bit. If there is any tension lingering around, take a big inhale through your nose and long exhale out through your mouth. Twice more just like that. When you're ready, rest here.

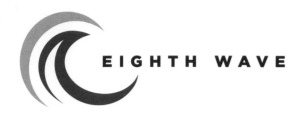

EIGHTH WAVE

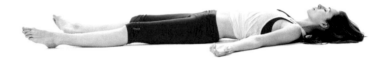

Here you have an opportunity to connect with several people through touch. It's a great time to be silent. Make your way around the room to support people with touch when appropriate.

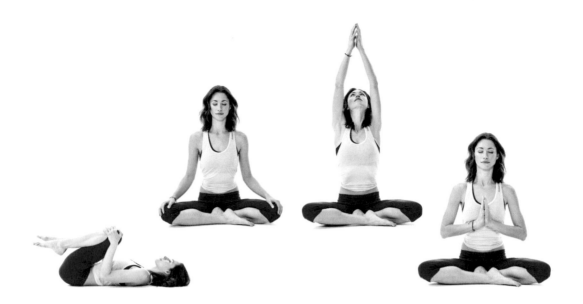

It's great to be in the front of the room, sitting easily, as you guide people to come out of the relaxation and meeting them in easy seated for meditation.

Start to invite some more air back into your body. Roll around your wrists and ankles if that feels nice. Stretch out your arms overhead if that feels nice. When you're ready, hug your knees into your chest, and make your way up to sit in the easiest way.

Close your eyes and let your attention drift inward. Take a big inhale and float your arms up and overhead. Press your palms together and bring your thumbs to your heartbeat. Soften here for a moment. Take a big inhale through your nose. Exhale out through your mouth. Twice more like that, big inhale. Long exhale. One more time, big inhale, long exhale. Soften here for a moment.

<h1 style="text-align:center">Namaste and thank you
for coming!</h1>

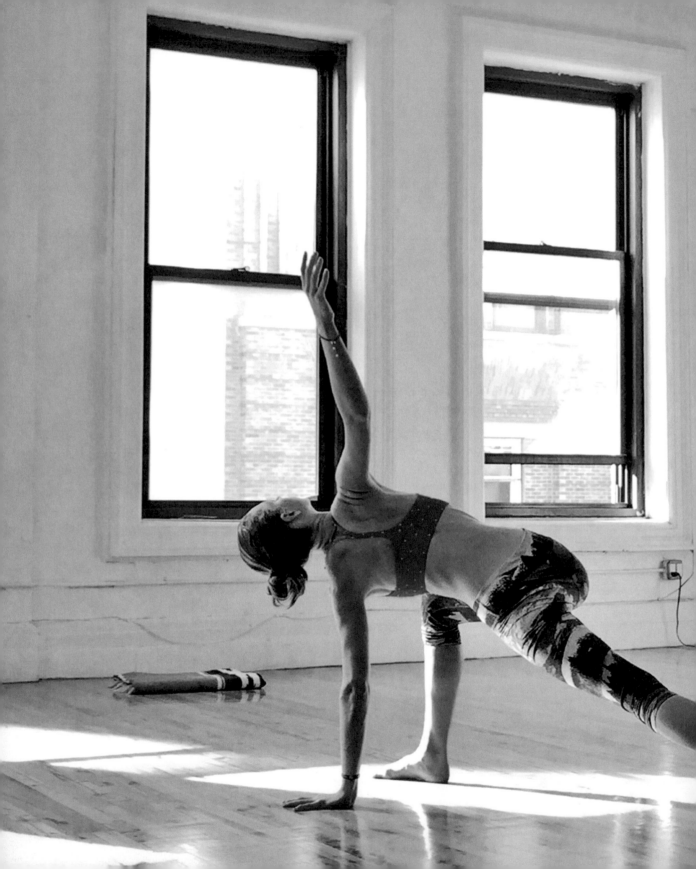

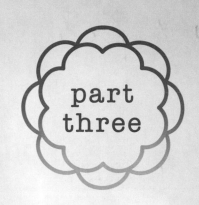

part
three

beyond yoga

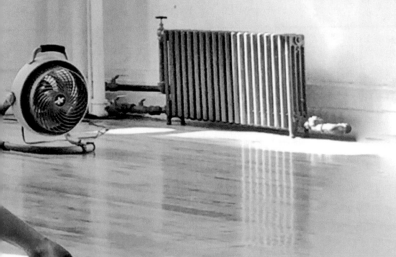

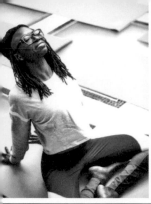

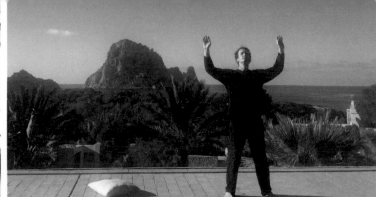

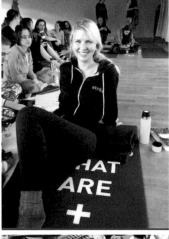

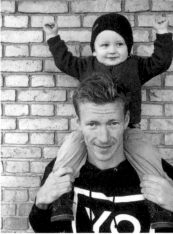

> **"**
>
> You might find that going easy on yourself is the best way to do everything there is.
>
> **"**

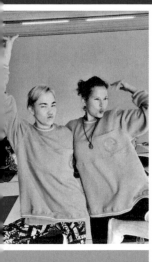

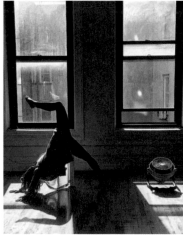

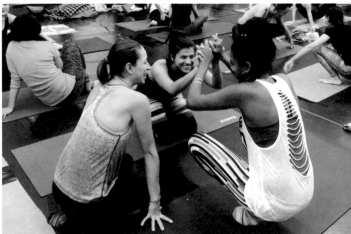

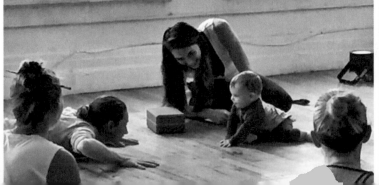

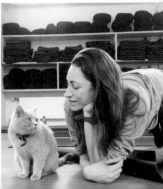

NOURISHING BODY & SOUL

EMBODYING A HEALTHY LIFESTYLE

An amazing transformation happens when you become a yoga teacher or, in our case, a Guide. You are assumed to be an expert in pretty much everything wellness. From food to relationships to wardrobe to finances to life choices, you'll be bombarded with all sorts of questions from people who come to your classes and want to connect with you in other ways. It's a wonderful privilege and important responsibility to treat people with respect and kindness and to offer support, useful knowledge, and suggestions when appropriate.

You might be the first to know about a pregnancy—sometimes even before a partner—or you might be confided in when someone is dealing with an eating disorder, death in the family, life crisis, or sickness, or you may simply be asked for advice for dealing with everyday stresses. With the cardinal rule of "do no harm" as our governing principle, I urge you not to play

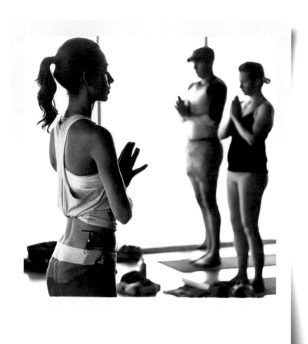

doctor, psychologist, or family member, unless you do have that appropriate relationship with the person asking.

With regard to nourishment, stress, and helping people create a sustainable, enjoyable lifestyle, where they can function freely in their lives, it's useful to know that our job of guiding the class is aimed at dissolving stress from the body and mind. Stress is our number one cause of food issues. Overeating, undereating, controlled eating, disorders, and stress eating all fall under the category of "stress." Use your common sense and intuition when advising someone on their diet. So much can be accomplished by helping people dissolve stress through the experience you provide.

Food has a whole lot to do with *how you feel* about food and only a little to do with what you are actually eating. When we balance how we feel, balancing our eating becomes easy.

When we get together in groups for training and talk about food, diet, and stress, it's always a passionate, intense, and wonderfully diverse conversation. We bring up the topic of food and how it relates to guiding and advising others. But I love to open the conversation to something more personal—asking about personal relationships to food and if anyone has noticed any differences in how they feel and eat since we have been together. The feedback is often dramatic and incredibly unique for each person. Some people report being hungrier and needing more food to sustain themselves throughout the day. Some report being less hungry and eating more simple and nutrient-dense foods, like smoothies, to gain energy for the day. Many report being more sensitive to their food choices, and craving more nourishing foods and enjoying eating more than before. This is all from just a few days of intense practice. Lots of people report changes with wants and needs when it comes to sugar and caffeine. Most say they crave less coffee and sugar and end up having loads more energy. Many people say they are sleeping better and feel more energized. They also report that their digestion is working better than usual. Some eat plant-based diets, some are omnivores, and some maintain other diets. The point is, before we began practice, no suggestion about food was necessary. The practice of sensitizing ourselves to how our bodies and minds feel with the class is enough to put us on the path to well-being. This happens on a chemical and emotional level.

SENSITIZE YOURSELF TO THE RIGHT FOOD CHOICES FOR YOU

We all know that we should eat more plants and fresh foods and fewer processed foods. We know we should cook more at home and eat on the run less. Knowing what to do isn't what stops us from making better choices. It's often priorities and stress that come into action. Everyone is insanely busy. The food industry caters to our packed schedules, making it simple to pick up anything on the run. The problem is that the fast pickup options are never the healthy ones. They leave us feeling not great and desiring more quick fixes. Thus perpetuating the unhealthy cycle. Hopefully we wake up before sickness enters the picture.

The more we practice taking care of ourselves with easygoing yoga and meditation, the more we are inclined to continue that self-care when we leave the practice room. This seeps over into our food choices, relationships, work choices, and in general, how we feel about pretty much everything. Sensitizing is the real deal, and it's useful that you understand its power for yourself and when advising others.

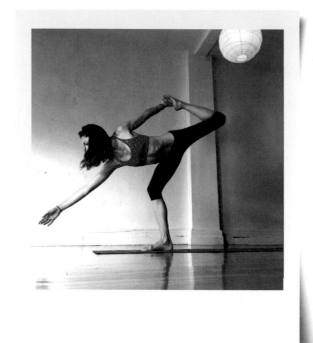

What we can help people with is dissolving stress, connecting back to self, and spending time in a positive community. The act of getting together for practice is good practice for getting together with people in the rest of life. Spending time with your friends and family cooking in the kitchen is one of the healthiest practices we can have around how we feel about food. Also when we prepare our own meals, we know better what we are consuming and where it comes from. We are also waging a pretty powerful protest against big food companies that set out to control every aspect of our eating and feed us the cheapest products possible—things that are destructive not only to our health and well-being but also to our community and planet.

WHEN FOLLOWING HOW YOU FEEL DOESN'T WORK

Sensitizing with the practice works when the individual is within a healthy range of mental and physical health. When we are faced with someone in an extreme situation, like someone who has a severe anxiety disorder or eating disorder, guiding them to follow how they feel would be guiding them deeper into their imbalance. When it "feels good" for a person to behave unhealthily, there is a need for concern and possibly intervention by referral to a specialist. Unless you are a medical doctor, don't play doctor when people come to you with serious health issues. With cases of severe eating disorders, we are careful to listen to the person if she wants to talk, encourage her to participate in gentle classes instead of more athletic ones that require more energy and can feed the disorder, and in some cases, reach out to family members to voice concern. It's a sensitive issue when someone is imbalanced, but always remember, our main concern needs to be that person's safety. The easygoing movements can be very healing and have done wonders for many people suffering from disorders, but we must be careful when giving advice.

I have a circle of experts and professionals in the health field I trust and use as referrals. I suggest you do the same. And be prepared to advise people to back off, slow down, and take it easy. It's a great step if someone with a disorder is there to attend your class. Depending on whether you own the studio or are working for a studio or gym, you might feel compelled to have a conversation with the management about the person to decide together how it is most appropriate to help the person in need. Ignoring a problem in this case is not a good solution. If someone is able to walk through the door for class, he is able to be helped on some level by you. If you feel unable to address the situation and it makes you uncomfortable or nervous, enlist the help of your co-workers privately in conversation, so you feel more prepared when the person visits. These situations aren't fun, but know that you being present with the person can often make a major difference in his or her life. You have the power to affect positive change with your attention.

THE SCIENCE OF NUTRITION, MOOD & HEALTH
Getting into Your Microbiome

We can't address our health, food, and nutrition without first looking at stress, and how we feel in our bodies each day. Strala has been carefully designed to support us in the path we all need to self-connection, sensitizing us to how we feel, and responding to this feeling each day, in how we move through our lives. It's our first key to letting the stress go and becoming our own best caregivers.

There's one more key here, hidden inside each of us. It's as unique as you are, and it plays a central role in digestion, metabolism, and appetite. It's also a primary factor in your mood and mental acuity and heart and bone health, is critical to your immunity, and even produces natural antibiotics. It's called your microbiome: a community of bacteria that lives in each of us. These bacteria outnumber our own cells by a factor of 10 to 1—you're carrying about 100 trillion of them right now—and they have co-evolved to a critical role in supporting our health and well-being.

An unhealthy microbiome can lead to frequent colds, muscle and joint pain, unneeded weight gain, fatigue, anxiety, and depression, as well as leaky gut and an associated cascade of allergies. So what makes our microbiome unhealthy? Stress is a big factor here, and it can unbalance our microbiome in a single day. Medications, including antibiotics and NSAIDs, infection, and inflammation all play damaging roles. And, finally, food is a big element. Sugar, animal fats, and alcohol all create an environment that favors the bacteria we don't want and limits the ones we do.

It's also important to recognize the role of our microbiome in unhealthy weight gain. When our gut is healthy, it produces short-chain fatty acids (SCFAs)

that signal when we are full and lead to faster digestion, which means less calorie extraction. This production falls off when our microbiome isn't properly balanced. We've known for decades that we can make cows fat by subjecting them to loads of stress and filling them with low levels of microbiome-harming antibiotics. Now we're just beginning to talk about the same impact on humans, and it's vital to get to the word out. Stress and the balance of our microbiome form the two most significant factors in obesity, for both children and adults.

The good news is we can change our microbiome. The big first step is to release stress from our bodies and minds, by learning how to move easily—with grace and coordination—in everything we do. This reduces inflammation and creates the environment we want for a happy microbiome. From here, there's a host of foods, known as prebiotics, that move things along in the right direction. Put lots of variety in your everyday choices, including fermented foods, whole foods, and plenty of fruits and vegetables, including fiber. Of course, we already know these things are good for us. Now we know even more just how powerful the choices we make really are.

ADVISING BY EXAMPLE

Our health is multifaceted. Sleep, relaxation, activity, practice, nourishment, stress, purpose, relationships, work, family—these factors interconnect and contribute to our well-being. It's hard to guide them all, but the best way we can is to live it. We need to radiate a healthy, honest lifestyle of attainable well-being by practicing sensitizing regularly ourselves. I've made it a mission of mine to create, discover, and improvise healthy, easy-to-make recipes that are inexpensive. Health shouldn't be available only to people who can afford to shop at expensive markets and have tons of free time to cook. Because of my personal mission, I am able to connect and share with people about all these fun, delicious, healthy, and inexpensive recipes. I've chosen not to preach about a specific diet but cook with mostly plants and simple ingredients. I reason that if I can encourage people to cook at home more, buy simple, unprocessed foods, and throw them together in the kitchen creatively, that is a great and sustainable practice for our well-being.

You can invent your own version of what you care about with food, and you probably are already doing this. The secret is to share when it's natural with those who come to your classes and to involve cooking and eating as a community endeavor, whether you are having potlucks at your place once a month or swapping recipes here and there.

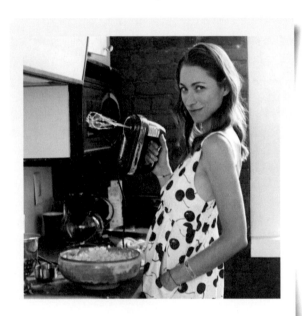

The idea is to create excitement around inventing, creating, and enjoying cooking and eating well. When we enjoy and feel like we are creating instead of following the rules or a diet, we take ownership of what we cook and eat, and are on our way to sustainable, radiant well-being. Isn't that exciting!

Just like the classes you're leading, people do what you do, not what you say, so when you're in a position of influence, it's important to be a good example for yourself and for those you're aiming to help. So get involved in the process instead of being prescriptive, and you'll enjoy having a small part to do with the well-being success of a wide range of people.

I've got three simple things you can do to help yourself and the people you serve to achieve radiant well-being. Ready? Let's go!

1. **GET INTERESTED.** Get interested in the people around you. How do they feel about food? Listen to them. Listen to what they say about their day. Are they stressed, tired, and worn-out? Are they feeling good and energized? The more you listen, the more you'll learn and be able to help.

2. **GET IN THE KITCHEN.** Roll up your sleeves. Get to the farmer's market and stock up on fresh produce and foods. Experiment and see what happens. Feed yourself and those around you.

3. **SHARE AND ENJOY!** Whether it's through dinner parties or sharing recipes in person, share your favorite recipes with those around you. Digital sharing is okay, but make sure it happens in person too. Get together with people regularly and cook. Swap ideas. Try things out. Keep connected to your community and watch it expand and gain radiant health. Enjoy!

Success is being able to spend
most of your time doing
what makes your whole self
come alive.

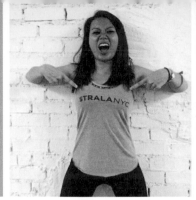
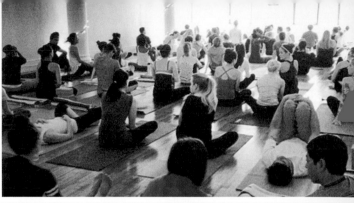
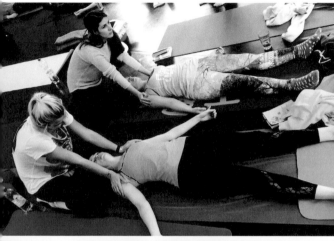
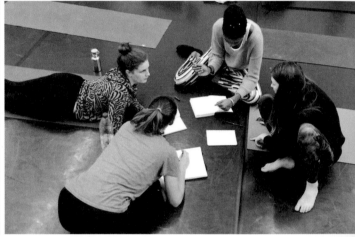
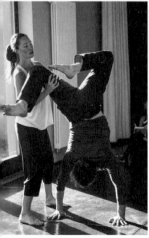

> "
> Put your attention
> on how you are.
> It creates who you are,
> which creates everything.
> "

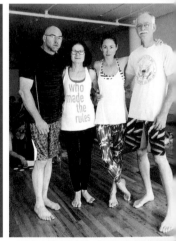
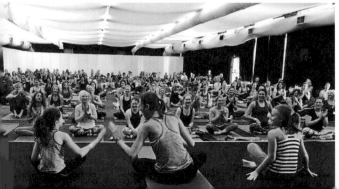
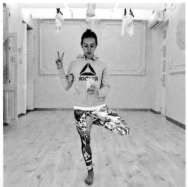

chapter
11

MINDFUL BUSINESS

TURNING YOUR PASSION
INTO YOUR WORK

Evolving your practice into a sustainable way to support yourself is a wonderful and worthy endeavor achievable through work and dedication. Beginning a business with the intention to help is something we need more of in this world. But it takes more than simply knowing how to guide people through a routine to create business.

A GUILTY EXCHANGE (OF MONEY)

The first part of making "Guide" be your job is to get over the guilt and self-doubt that often accompany accepting money for this work. It took me *years* before I felt okay with people paying in exchange for yoga help. Guiding people through this amazing process was just so emotional for me. It was something so special and sacred that I thought it was unreasonable to take money in exchange for sharing it. These feelings of self-doubt and guilt around money are common as you transition from simply working a job to pursuing a passion, so we need to heal them before we go about some of the more external practices that take us in the direction of our dreams. It's a bummer to have guilt and shame overshadow our hearts, skills, passions, drives, and talents for becoming an excellent Guide. You must learn that it is okay to accept money for doing something you love.

I led people one-on-one in their homes and in lots of group classes before I realized this. And I may not have realized it if it hadn't been for one person calling me out on it. She and I had worked together regularly for years, and she credited me for a great deal of her weight loss, getting off some medications, and simply feeling better. She was the one who told me I should be charging for my time. At the time I had other work; I didn't need yoga to be my income, so I saw no need to charge for it. But she reminded me that I could help even more people if I did this more full time rather than simply in my free time. She had a point. So I said, "I suppose I could charge $40 for an hour session." She laughed at me and said that her manicurist charges more for an hour. I said, "You must have very important nails." This just shows what a problem I had in this realm. I decided that I needed to think about it for a bit and make some decisions on how to move forward.

While I liked my other job, helping people through yoga really got me excited. I loved it. So why shouldn't I spend more of my time doing it? I settled for the moment on $60 per hour for the people I was seeing privately in their homes. And crazily enough, they were all thrilled that I was finally charging. Within a month I started earning enough from those one-on-one sessions to pay my bills. The people I had been working with all had friends and referrals that wanted in now that I had more availability. I was seeing several people a day for private classes and became superbusy doing what I loved. This happened gradually, then suddenly, with years of practice, and I have to admit, today with all the growth of Strala, and with the global network of Guides and studios and partnerships, I feel just as rewarded as the moment I realized I was able to pay my bills by helping people.

Before you can start creating a life in which you can sustain yourself financially doing something you love, you have to accept that it's okay to be paid for the service you're providing. Yes, you love guiding. Yes, you love living with ease. Yes, you love helping people. Because you love it, you likely can't imagine getting paid for it. We've been led to believe that work must be hard. That we must push and force our way through pain in order to be rewarded. But this isn't the case. You must remember that you are on a path that will help people live a happier, fuller life. They couldn't necessarily do that without you, so they will be happy to pay for it. It's a win-win situation. Everyone gets happy. So if you feel any guilt or self-doubt when you're doing this, look at your intentions. Be clear on why you're doing this. If helping people doesn't get you charged up, you're probably going in the wrong direction.

SUSTAINING YOUR BUSINESS

When I set about creating my business, I needed to figure out some simple, attainable goals that would be sustainable. As part of that, I came up with some clear priorities of how I wanted to run things. Just like the practice itself, I was focused on the process, not the end result. I wanted to tap into how I felt as I did things, and I wanted to make sure that the moves I made were in my long-term best interest. Basically I immersed myself in the process of creating my business. I had no idea how big it would get. That was never my focus. I simply wanted to help people, and by sticking with my priorities, I was able to go way beyond my goals—with less effort, moving through the challenges with ease.

Here are the things I focused on in my process—just so you can draw from them as you create your own process. Stick to these, and you'll find yourself on the way to a sustainable business.

PRIORITIZE IMPROVING

Just like the practice, you're never done. When we get into the mind-set of all the boxes are checked, and I've got this, we leave no room to grow. All the best Guides and leaders consistently practice. There is no limit on how easy you can make a challenge in your practice, or how much you can harness the breath and feeling in relation to the flow. The more you practice, the more you will understand in your own experience, so you can relate better to others.

Be constructively critical with yourself when it comes to your practice as well as to your leading. What and how could you have done better? When someone doesn't enjoy my class, I always ponder what I could have done to support her better. Every time I lead a class, event, workshop, or training, I allow myself time for reflection for improvement, and I ask some people for critical feedback. It's not appropriate to ask this of people who come for your classes, but you can develop a relationship with other Guides or other people who are willing to play this role for you. For the average class participant, you'll know if they liked it or not based on if they come back. By the time you are leading classes, you should be able to identify what went right and what you can improve on. Between that and some occasional input from your network of Guides, you can create a better and better experience.

In trainings we encourage critical feedback when people partner up to learn and practice the elements of leading. When you're on your way to guiding for money, make sure to find someone who will be picky with you. You won't learn much about yourself if your partner dares only to say, "That was nice." A useful conversation feels more like this, "I liked the place you chose to touch me in pigeon, but I felt like you didn't bring your whole self to the situation," or "The pressure was superficial and not a relaxed lean." Or "Your demonstrating and mirroring in class were really great, but I couldn't hear you all the time. Maybe breathing deeper while leading will help everyone hear you clearly." We can give this kind of feedback to ourselves, as well. Keeping an improvement journal is a great idea. I have one. I also often ask Mike and Sam for feedback, as well as some of the Guides I've known for a long time. It's a useful practice to get comfortable with.

We offer several programs for education, intensives, long trainings, and continuing education. There are many successful Guides who complete only one intensive and many who complete longer trainings and who take longer to embody the concepts and gain experience leading. One training schedule doesn't fit all, but it's important to continue to improve your skills with real-world practice leading, and come back occasionally when you have questions and feel a wall approaching. Always keeping the mind of a student and a beginner will help you improve rapidly when you return for education. I love seeing you again in the programs, but even more I love seeing you succeed in your careers.

CREATE & ACCEPT OPPORTUNITIES

This is an idea that really takes you to the next level in your business: spend time accepting opportunities that come your way, as well as creating opportunities where you see none. If you do this on a regular basis, you will eventually have more opportunities than you have time for. This can happen quickly—as in a few months—or more gradually over the course of a couple of years. Whatever the timeline, building a fulfilling life based around passion is fluid, and you have to just go with the flow. Your life this month will probably be very different from your life a year from now. Where you lead, who you connect and partner with, and what tools you use to communicate your services will all evolve. Just like the practice, we achieve more when we are soft and easygoing. Avoid becoming rigid in what you believe your life should look like day to day. Keep yourself open to opportunity, and your schedule will fill up before you can take three deep breaths. It's not magic; it's simply about where you put your energy and how great it feels.

So let's talk about opportunity and creating them where you see none. Entering into the world as a Guide, you are an entrepreneur. If this idea is overwhelming or scary, there are plenty of viable options for things you can do while you get comfortable with it. Look for a full-time job leading at a health club or an established yoga studio. Or even work toward being program director or manager at one of these places. There are lots of Guides who create wonderful, sustainable lives earning their livings by being employees of a company that embodies their passions. Leading classes at other companies is also a wonderful option that many businesses are interested in. The word kind of got out that yoga and meditation have a direct effect on well-being, which means fewer sick days and increased productivity, focus, and creativity.

I'm a card-carrying member of the insane entrepreneurs of the world club. It's not better to be working for yourself, or better to find peace in being an employee. I believe it's programmed into how we all are, with some flexibility on what we gravitate toward with our life experience and tolerance. So please don't beat yourself up or think something is wrong if you are more comfortable one way or the other. Both are great, valuable, and worthy.

If you enjoy being on your own and creating your own opportunities, there are lots that aren't visible until you create them. I started free yoga in Central Park. After a while I created some YouTube videos, I blogged, and I led one-on-one classes. These things led to the addition of an apartment studio, which I eventually made more legit by moving into a commercial studio, where I could grow some roots. One thing doesn't necessarily lead to the next and the next in a linear fashion, but things work out quickly when you take and create many opportunities at once. Doing only one thing at a time is a much slower process that has a higher chance of leading only to itself and eventually a dead end. Lead everywhere you can, and you'll be leading full time soon.

On the topic of money, this is a bit more of an individual choice, but I have some suggestions based in personal experience and what I've seen work and not work in the real world. Full disclosure, I still do things for free all the time. I lead some privates for free, based on need, certain events, especially those for a good cause, and I collaborate on projects based on how I feel more than what the financial return is. We keep drop-in classes and workshop prices affordable, and our trainings are well below the cost of average trainings, which are often led by people with little experience. We could charge a lot more and get away with it, but it's not in my value system. A big part of my mission is to provide great, quality products at an affordable cost. I don't want people to have to choose between a yoga class and buying quality produce. That's just not going to benefit the world.

It's important to charge a fair price for your work but not value yourself so much that you lose integrity and create an unsustainable situation for those you are serving. There are gobs of yoga teachers and trainers out there charging 10 times what we charge, but I believe it's unethical and puts a heavy layer of dependence on the student-teacher relationship. When Guides we train are fresh and dive into leading classes and workshops charging more than we do, they aren't my first to elevate and suggest as a good example of self-value or standards. Aim to price your work so it's sustainable for you, and sustainable for those who choose to practice with you.

If you are working for a studio, it's more realistic to ask for a low base fee and a bonus per person over a certain amount of people in your classes rather than a flat fee that may be more than the income your class brings in. Allowing yourself to be rewarded for bringing people into the studio will be sustainable for the owner and motivate you to do a good job and also invite people into the space. Gyms and clubs usually have different policies regarding flat fees, but they might be able to give you more classes per week to lead than an independent studio. There is a third option, which is my personal favorite. Rent a by-the-hour space that is convenient for people to come to and start to build your local community. Charge a fair and reasonable price in relation to how much experience you have leading, and enjoy how you can create exactly the environment you want—and the reward of keeping the income the class brings. This is more risky, of course. What if no one shows, and you're stuck with the rental fee for the hour? But hey, that's great motivation to communicate to everyone you meet about your classes. The more you talk about what you do and where it's available, the more likely you are to succeed. If you're shy about it and don't tell anyone, you'll be sitting alone with a nice bill to pay.

BRING YOUR WHOLE SELF TO THE SITUATION

There is no exit strategy for me, no endgame. I just want to live a life of integrity and help people. I want to focus on the process of doing this. I have the pleasure of speaking on panels about business, and I've come to realize that this isn't how most businesses are run. People start companies now to get out of them in five years. People work so they can get rich and stop working. My goal has always been to help people. I can't imagine not doing this. It *is* me—which means that I bring my whole self to my business. It's not a job—it's me.

Not surprisingly to me, other people and companies who apply this way of thinking achieve lots of success, both monetarily and in the health of their businesses and its leaders. Focusing on the process over the goal propels you far past your goal with ease. This works for natural movement in practice and in business. Pretty great, right? We are literally practicing this in class. While we sensitize ourselves, we are practicing being good at living, good at business, good at leading, and good at being.

This is about helping people and freeing up my time and energy constantly in a way that best serves that mission. It was the same mission then as it is now.

The secret to having a sustainable business is walking into the open doors of opportunity always with the aim to help. There are always people in this world who will need help, so you'll always have something to do. You might not be entitled to earn your living in your first year or several years of leading, but if you stay with your practice, improve your skills with experience, and keep your intentions honorable with the people you interact and work with, you'll have more opportunities than you can accept. I promise you.

CREATING YOUR LIFE

creating your life circle

Circle requires regular practice & action.
Doesn't work if you don't do it.

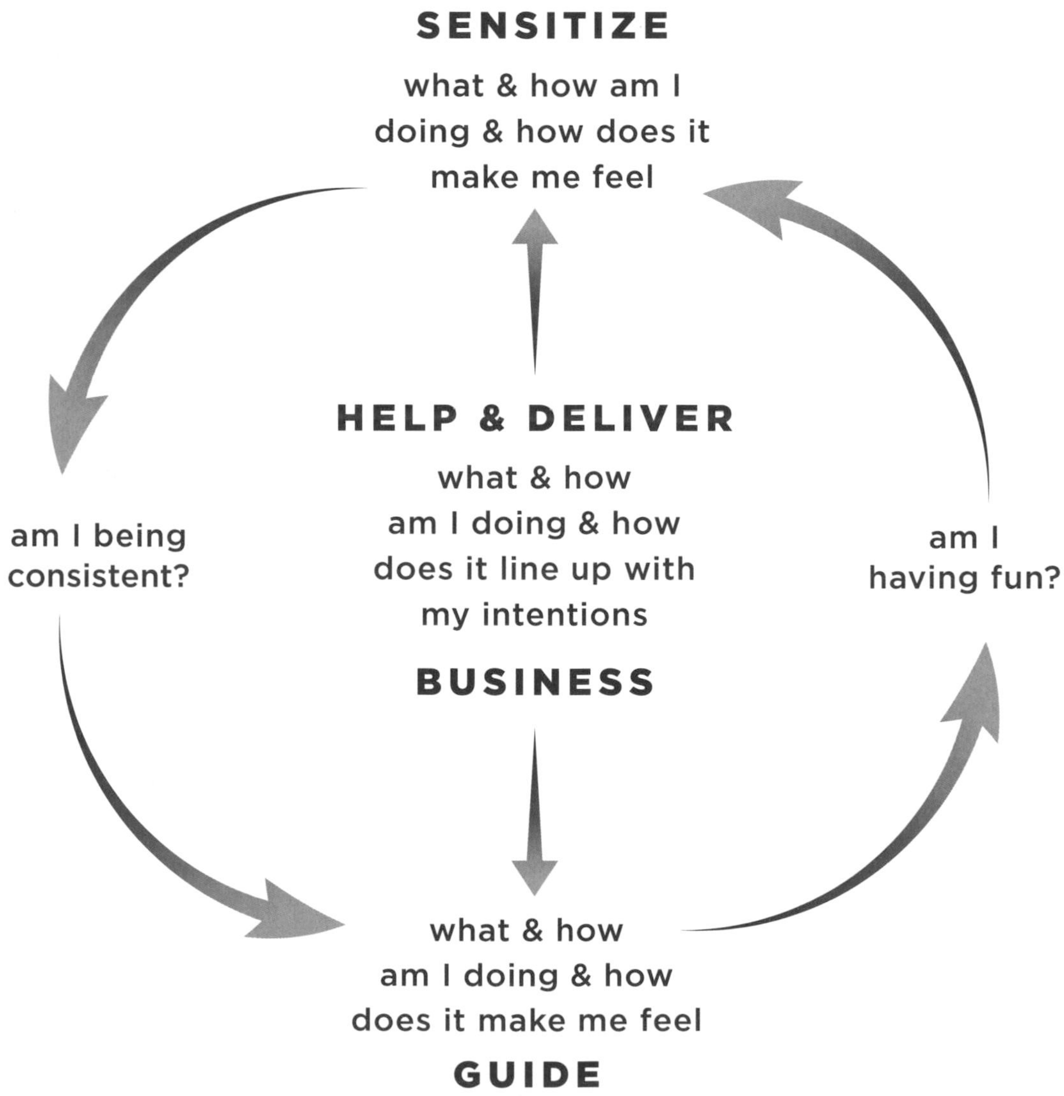

SENSITIZE

what & how am I
doing & how does it
make me feel

HELP & DELIVER

what & how
am I doing & how
does it line up with
my intentions

am I being
consistent?

am I
having fun?

BUSINESS

what & how
am I doing & how
does it make me feel

GUIDE

There is a lovely circle of factors to consider that can help you think about what you aim to build and how to create this life for yourself sustainably. These are the pieces of creating and sustaining the life you're working to build, along with some questions to ask yourself as you consider the direction you're moving in.

SENSITIZE: At the top of the circle, we have sensitize. Everything comes back to following how we feel. We know we share what we have, so our main job is self-practice and self-care.

GUIDE: What am I doing, and how does it make other people feel? We need to ask ourselves this as we step into the role of the Guide. We listen to others instead of going on and on about ourselves. We observe with consideration and with an eye and an ear to help. We practice our skills, aiming to improve so we can help more effectively. We acknowledge that we have a lifetime of practice ahead, and we enjoy getting better at what we do.

HELP AND DELIVER: Our intentions are like a flashlight we use to navigate our path home on a dark night. Without our intentions, we become lost, have a hard time focusing and making decisions, and run the risk of becoming depressed about our career choice, which leads to fatigue and lack of motivation. With a proper intention, we are fueled up, light shining brightly showing the path all the way home. We are able to enjoy the journey because we are safe, on a well-lit path, and able to make decisions about what to do and which way to go. When carving out your own career, every moment is a decision that could change your life. Come back to your intentions when you have a doubt and you'll be guided in the right direction.

Ask yourself, "What am I doing, and is it in line with my intentions?" Your intention may be as simple as "I want to help people feel better." Or as specific as "I want to help people overcome trauma." If your intention is "I want to be famous and make a lot of money," please put this book down and go directly to volunteer at a homeless shelter until your attitude shifts.

CONSISTENCY: This is a more technical and important consideration for what you are doing. Are you offering a public class? Is it at a regular time in a convenient location? Do you show up regularly and deliver a quality experience? Do you communicate through digital means or flyers or meet people in person to find opportunities to lead? Do you wait to be invited for opportunities or do you create your own? Do you take the reins to offer a studio owner a free sample

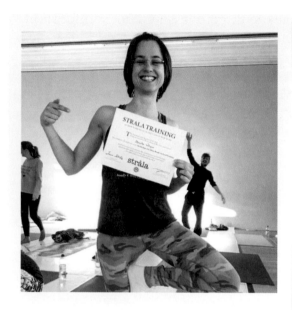

class, or rent a space by the hour to hold a class a few times a week? Are you giving a weekly class outdoors in the summer to make it easy for people to get to know you? Do you say yes to opportunity easily, or do you take a lot of time to consider what you are going to get out of the situation?

FUN: Just like our principles of movement, fun is critical to your success. So ask yourself if you're enjoying what you're doing or feel like you're trudging along to reach a goal. Do you believe you'll be happy when certain things might happen in the future or are you happy with what you have right now? Do you enjoy leading and working with people? If you're having fun, you're in a good place. If you're not having fun, look at all the things you're doing and see what changes you can make. If you're having fun, you'll enjoy sustainable bursts of energy to support your efforts. Just like in practice. Funny how the practice, the philosophy, the lifestyle, and the business are all the same, isn't it? So let's have some fun helping people and enjoy having a small part to do with their success and a bigger part to do with yours.

By keeping these five factors in mind as you're developing your business—and occasionally asking yourself these questions even after you've had some success—you'll create something that you enjoy and can sustain for years to come. The details and questions that might otherwise cause worry as you go out into the world and create new opportunities become simple logistics that are fun to navigate. When you come back to the process and, most important, prioritize being the example of what you'd like to help others with, you'll surprise yourself, just like in our physical practice of going much further than you might have ever thought possible when working with efficiency, natural movement, grace, and ease. Your success has no limits when you align with yourself, continue to improve, and lead with the intention to help and serve.

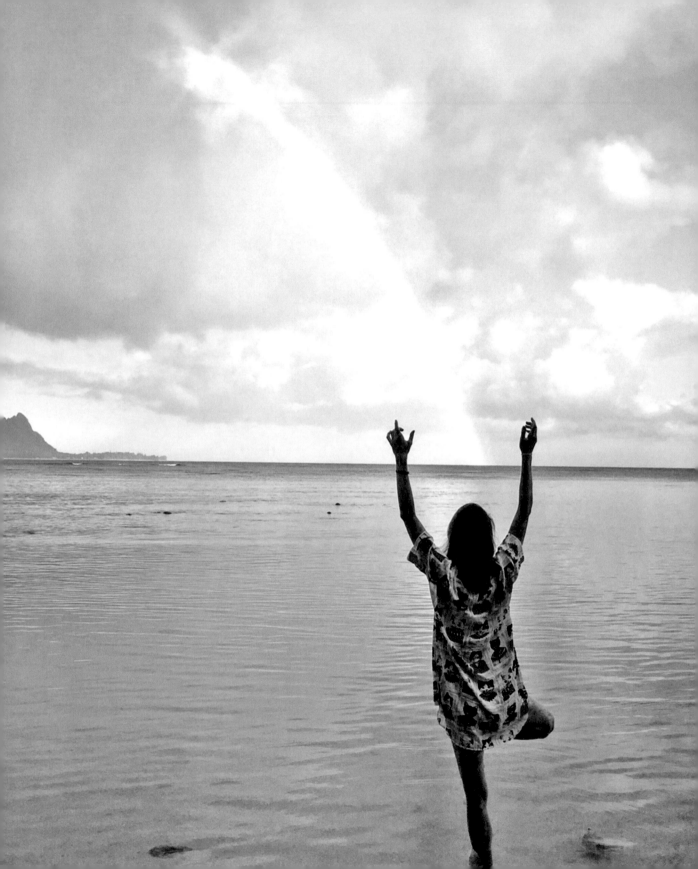

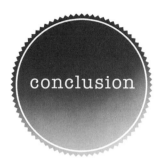

conclusion

FINAL WISHES FOR YOU

Healing is what Strala is all about. It's about creating a life of ease that leads to joy, health, and well-being. When we soften, breathe, move from the middle, and connect with those around us from this place, we find magic. We thrive in our connection to each other and with ourselves.

Every moment is an opportunity for change. You are part of that change. By living as an example of ease and love, you can change the world around you—and the change will ripple into the world at large. It's amazing what we can do when we stand together against difficulty, stress, pressure, and hate.

While you may not be able to see your effect on the bigger picture, you can see it in the people who come to you for help. One of my favorite stories is from a woman named Christine, whose life was truly shifted by the practice of ease.

CHRISTINE:

I've lived in Berkeley, California, since 1991, when I was an undergrad at UC Berkeley. This is a land with no lack of incense, tie-dyed T-shirts, and yoga studios, but I didn't find yoga here; I found yoga while living in New York City 20 years later when, in the most timid of manners, I stepped into a RELAX class at Strala with my friend.

We just wanted to get moving. We were both writers who sat at desks all day. We would never describe ourselves as athletic or coordinated. We both hated exercise classes; I disliked them because I felt so self-conscious in a classroom setting, where my place in the spectrum (worst in class) would be so marked. But we thought it would be good to get more flexible. We picked the studio because, in all frankness, it was conveniently located. In sum, we had no expectations.

But there we were, with Tara, who would occasionally giggle to herself and bring laughter into the room. Because of this, I began to equate yoga with delight. She welcomed us as if into her own home, and didn't make me feel like a failure because I struggled to hold downward dog those first weeks. It was okay. I went back the next week. And then the next. I upped my visits to two times a week, sometimes three over the next year.

What happened over the next year and a half at Strala Yoga was life changing.

But in order to tell you what changed, I feel like I should tell you a little about my relationship with my body: I have had a painful relationship with my body—in fact, I wanted to divorce myself from my body. It had let me down in so many ways that I'd assumed it would always disappoint me. I was not nice to my body, either—I starved it, I purged it, and I hurt myself in retaliation and in pursuit of control throughout my teenage years.

In my late 20s, I was diagnosed with polycystic ovary syndrome (PCOS). It was undiagnosed until a few years after my husband and I tried to conceive. When I saw my ovaries on the ultrasound, my first reaction was, "They look like a pomegranate cross section!" They were filled with dozens of unpopped eggs, cysts if you will. I cried when I found out—not from grief but from relief. I had finally found a name for what was wrong with my body. I found out that I'd been chubby and sluggish and moody not out of lack of discipline but because of a hormonal imbalance. I cried because I was angry that I'd gone undiagnosed for all those years, and because the side effects of PCOS (easy weight gain, difficult weight loss) could have been mitigated. I had engaged in needless war with my body and with myself.

And so I had renewed hope. I exercised. I ran. But you see, when I worked out, I was like a fainting goat. I'd run and want to pass out. Any strenuous weight lifting, and I'd go home with a migraine. I did stadium stairs, and I'd vomit 14 times in an hour. My personal trainer high-fived me for pushing through the pain each time.

I love backpacking. I've backpacked the Lost Coast, and I've backpacked throughout the Sierra Nevada mountains at altitude. My friends and I got used to the fact that I got altitude sickness before everyone else and that I'd just puke my way up the mountain.

And then I had a stroke in December 2006 at the age of 33 due to a PFO, which is a patent foramen ovale, a hole in the center of my heart. As fetuses, we breathe through our mothers' blood, and so we have no use for our lungs. The blood flows from one side of the heart to the other, skipping our lungs, through a hole in the central wall. When we start breathing air that hole is supposed to close and route blood to our lungs, but in about 20 percent of us, it remains open to varying degrees. A small percentage of us have migraines due to that hole, and an even smaller percentage can have a stroke. On December 31, 2006, I threw a clot into my brain and had a left thalamic stroke, one that left me with a 15-minute short-term memory.

Doctors closed the hole in my heart a few months later. I was restricted from exercising until I healed. I couldn't read anything other than People magazine for months. I couldn't read a novel for a year. I couldn't write fiction for nearly two years.

And when my heart was ready a year later, I began running again, in earnest. I could run. I could breathe. I couldn't believe the freedom. There was still a lot of healing left to do—doctors are amazing, but after my stroke, I learned that medicine can only go so far; that last mile is a lonely road that doctors often do not take alongside you. My neurologist told me as his parting words, "You've come a long way. You're lucky to be alive. But this is as far as I can take you." He was a wonderful neurologist who said this with the greatest of empathy. But it was the truth. This was as far as he could take me. The rest was up to me. And I pushed forward. I wrote every day, hoping to regain my ability to write. And I did.

But you see, it wasn't until Strala and Tara that I finished healing, when everything came together, my mind, my body, that last mile. My relationship between my mind and body. It wasn't until Strala that I realized there shouldn't be pain in wellness. There should be ease. That this new ability to breathe could connect my mind with my body. That every breath could heal.

I spent a year not running. I thought, What if I just do yoga? What if I really just enjoy myself and my body? What if I slow down?

To reiterate, there was still a lot of healing left to do, stuff I didn't even expect to have healed—my husband and I were still struggling to have a child. I'd taken progesterone, taken fertility medications, lost weight, taken metformin therapy. It had been a 13-year-long road, one not without its share of "let's give up for a while," and "let's try this or that again," and "I guess our life would be fine if we didn't have a kid" conversations. I was approaching 40, and the door was closing.

In the meantime, I was going to Strala. In the beginning, I trembled during warrior 2, but I'd take a deep breath, think of water, think my body was floating in water, and exhale, transition to reverse warrior 2, breathe, exhale, back to warrior 2, forward to triangle. Breathe. Easy. Slow. Breathe. Tara's voice was in my head. Ease. Easy. Breathe. Slow.

I was going to Strala. Mostly RELAX but some STRONG. For me, yoga wasn't about doing inversions or balancing on one arm. It was about 90 minutes with myself.

I was going to Strala. I did crow. I couldn't believe that when the time came, I could balance my body on my knees. It took a breath, not force, to do so.

I was going to Strala. Where people like Mike Taylor say things like, "Move like you like yourself." I had begun to like myself. The war with my body had finally ceased.

I was going to Strala. Where change was happening every single minute. Without pain. Without struggle.

A work acquaintance of mine once told me, "Christine, if it were easy to be fit, everyone would be fit. Working out is supposed to be hard and painful." At the time I nodded. But today I'd shake my head. It doesn't have to be that way.

I happened to drop 15 more pounds over the course of my year at Strala. When I wasn't in New York, I popped in Tara's DVDs and did yoga at home. I happened to start eating better—not that I didn't eat my share of junk food, but I found myself having a few bites of chocolate and then stopping when I had my fill. So many things "happened to happen" with yoga that it can't be a coincidence.

And my backpacking didn't suffer, either, because I happened to become more aerobically fit—last fall, I found myself jogging up Sierra trails that I'd previously struggled to walk.

I happened to be happier. I happened to be more confident.

And this spring, I happened to become pregnant.

I didn't go into pregnancy without risks; I had had chronic high blood pressure for a number of years and was at risk for preeclampsia. The first thing doctors did was take me off blood pressure medications I'd been taking for 10 years. I was a little worried.

Every day during my pregnancy, I checked my blood pressure. It never went above 125/84. And on the days (and the day or two after) I did yoga, my blood pressure stayed at or below 115/75.

I happened to no longer need blood pressure medication. Without medications and with yoga, I happened to no longer have blood pressure as high as 160/120.

Yoga kept me and my kid safe throughout gestation. I happened to not have morning sickness. I happened to have a completely textbook pregnancy.

I'm now 38 weeks pregnant, a milestone I never thought I would reach. At this point in pregnancy, I'm uncomfortable but healthy, thanks to yoga. I did RELAX classes on DVD with a few modifications—no rocking on my belly—until the end of week 32, which in layman's speak is eightish months.

I did everything I could to get pregnant over the course of 13 years. I know deep in my heart that it was yoga that happened to be the variable of change. It was yoga that brought my body into balance—and I could see things become regular in a way that hadn't been before.

I'm not scared of labor, because I am going to go into it with the Strala Yoga philosophy of breathing and moving with ease. Because I now have faith in my body. And this—this is how Strala Yoga changed my life.

Isn't that amazing? Christine is the proud mother of a beautiful girl named Penny, who loves practicing yoga with her mom. You can change lives. Go forth with joy and passion and ease. Make the world a better place.

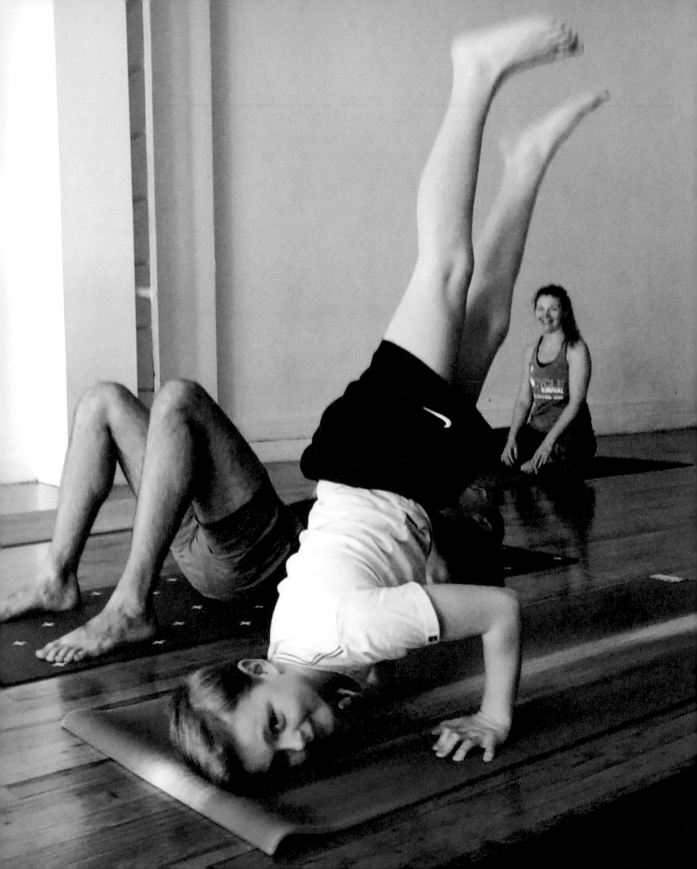

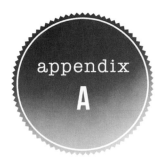

STRALA FOR CHILDREN

The following class is appropriate for most children ages 5 to 13. This can work in a mixed-age group, for an after-school or recess program, or at a studio or community center with a group.

    Taking the language of guiding into concern, when leading adult classes, the cuing of feeling is appropriately mature. Asking someone to follow how they feel, move how it feels good with the goal of sensitizing to themselves, is essential for adults but inappropriate for children. We wouldn't ask the children to move how it feels good, or to sensitize to themselves. Children gain wonderful benefits from yoga when they are guided clearly through the actions of the movements with the breath and allowed a natural sense of play within the class. Considering this point of view, we guide the action accompanied by the breath cue and lead groups of children into the movements by demonstrating, as well.

To see how language should change from adult to child, check out these two examples for instructing a move from standing to tree pose. The first is appropriate for adults.

> **Stand tall. Soften your knees and shift your weight onto your right leg. Hug your left shin in for a squeeze. Roll around in your hips how it feels good for you. When you're ready, come into your tree, placing your foot onto your thigh or on your ankle, however is most comfortable. Hang here for a few moments. Sway a bit side to side if that feels nice. When you're ready, give your shin a hug and softly place your foot back down coming into standing.**

And here is an appropriate guidance for children.

> **Stand tall. Bend your knees and shift your weight onto your right leg. Hug your left shin in for a squeeze. Open your knee out to the side and place the bottom of your foot onto your thigh or on your ankle, both are great. Thankfully all the trees are different, keeping the forest interesting. Reach your arms up and sway a bit in the breeze. Hug your shin back in toward you and place your foot down.**

Notice the slight difference between the two? We're very clear directionally with both versions, but instead of rolling around the hips how it feels good, we go right into the tree. We leave space for the children to get into the movement instead of asking them to come into it "whenever they feel ready." We say how all the trees are different, keeping the forest interesting, to avoid any problem of competition. Funny enough, this works great for adults, as well! I love to use it occasionally in my classes to help adults take the pressure off themselves. For the kids, it prevents hurt feelings, and bullying, celebrating the diversity we share with nature and harmony with the self.

Our goal of leading children is to support their abilities and to build confidence and body and mind awareness, while developing a healthy sense of self and community with a kindness and compassion. Many children are able to join adult classes, and it's best for the Guide and parent to use their best judgment on whether the child would enjoy the class, be able to move through the class without getting bored, and not be distracting to the rest of the participants. Usually children with a more athletic inclination are easy to integrate into adult classes starting at about age seven. It's important to remember that all children are different, just as all adults are different. Keep the child in mind when deciding if he or she is ready to participate in an adult class.

As always, stay easy, and enjoy!

STRALA KIDS

30-45 MINUTE CLASS EXAMPLE

This class has six waves instead of the eight waves we've been using in the other classes, supporting the length of time for the children's class. You can always adjust the class time by adding or subtracting waves or changing the length of the waves to support the time you have with your group.

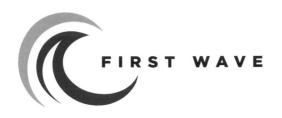

FIRST WAVE

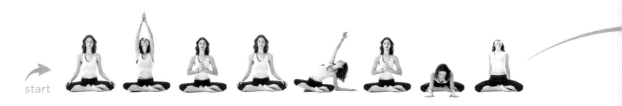

start

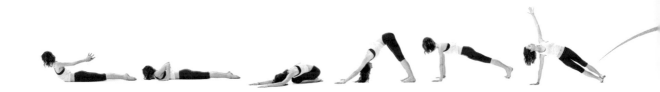

Demonstrate mirroring and facing the group to keep the rhythm and breath-body connection for the movements.

Sit comfortably. Take a big inhale and lift your arms out and up. Press your palms together and bring your thumbs to your heartbeat. Take a big inhale through your nose. Long exhale out through your mouth. Twice more like that. Big inhale. Long exhale. One more time. Big inhale. Long exhale. Relax your hands on your thighs and open your eyes.

Lean to your left and bring your left arm down toward the ground. Stretch your right arm up and overhead. Come back to the middle. Lean to your right and bring your right arm toward the ground. Reach your left arm up and overhead. Come back to the middle. Crawl yourself forward, walking your hands out in front of you. Relax your head and neck. Crawl yourself back up to your center. Bring your hands behind you on the ground. Press down through your hands, take a big inhale, and lift up. Exhale and come back to your center. Sit to your side, and come around onto all fours. Drop your belly and look upward. Round your back and look inward. We'll do that a few more times. Drop your belly and look upward. Round your back and look inward. One more time, drop your belly and look upward. Round your

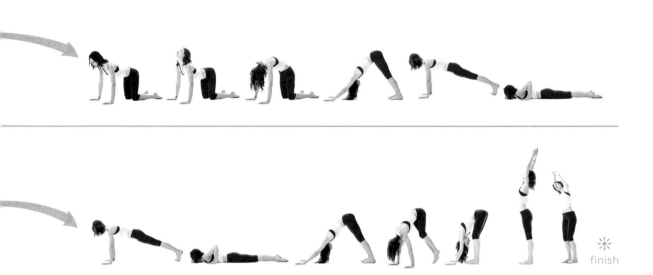

back and look inward. Drop your belly and look upward. Tuck your toes; lift your hips up and back to down dog. Relax your heels toward the ground and relax your head and neck. Tuck your chin and roll out to plank. Soften your elbows and lower to your belly. Interlace your hands behind you and lift up. Relax back to your belly. Press your palms to the ground and bring your hips to your heels for child's pose. Come back to all fours, tuck your toes, and lift up and back to down dog.

Tuck your chin and round back out to plank. Shift onto your right side and open up to your left for side plank. Come back to your center. Shift your weight on your left side, take a big inhale, and open to your right side. Come back to your center. Soften your elbows and lower to your belly. This time press right up and back to down dog.

Take a walk on up to the top of your mat. Relax your torso up and over your legs. Round up to stand one notch at a time. Once you make it up, reach your arms out and up. Grab hold of your left wrist with your right hand. Take a big inhale and lift up and over to your right. Come back to the center and grab hold of your right wrist with your left hand. Take a big inhale and lift up and over to your left. Come back to center.

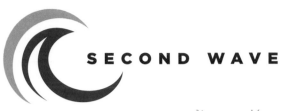

SECOND WAVE

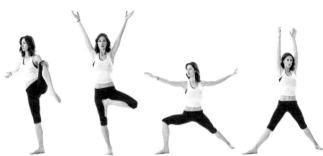

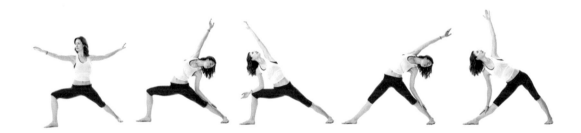

Shift your weight onto your right leg, hug your left shin into your chest. Bring the bottom of your foot onto your thigh so your knee points out. Reach your arms up. Stay easy here like a tree swaying in the breeze. Hug your shin into your chest and bring your foot back down.

Repeat on the other side.

Step your feet apart. Turn your right toes to point to your right and your left toes to turn in a bit so your heel faces out. Take a big inhale and open your arms out to your sides. Exhale and sink your hips, bending your front knee over your front foot. Look over your right hand and breathe here for three long, deep breaths. Take a big inhale and lift your hips and arms up overhead. Exhale back to warrior 2. Tip back to reverse warrior. Tip up and over extended side angle, bringing your right forearm to your thigh and arcing your left arm up and overhead. Press down through your legs, come back through warrior 2, and tip back to reverse warrior. This time tip back so much that your front leg straightens a bit. Tip up and over and bring your right hand to your right shin and open your left arm up for your triangle. Hang here for three long, deep breaths. Press down through your legs, take a big inhale, and come back up.

Swivel your toes around and we'll repeat on the other side.

THIRD WAVE

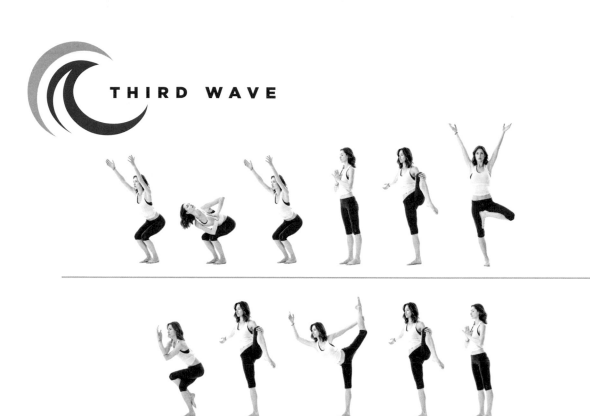

Bring your feet under your shoulders and stand up nice and tall. Bend your knees, sink your hips, and take a big inhale to lift up to chair pose. Bring your palms together and twist to your left. Take a big inhale and come back to chair. Twist to your right. Take a big inhale and come back to chair. Press down through your legs and come back to stand up tall.

Shift your weight onto your right leg; hug your left shin into your chest. Bring the bottom of your foot onto your thigh so your knee points out. Reach your arms up. Stay easy here like a tree, swaying in the breeze. Hug your shin into your chest and bring your foot back down.

Repeat on the other side.

Shift your weight onto your right leg; hug your left shin into your chest. Wrap your left leg around your right and your left arm under your right for your eagle pose. Sink through your hips and lift up through your fingertips. Unwind out and hug your left shin back into your chest. Place your foot back down.

Repeat on the other side.

Shift your weight onto your right leg; hug your left shin into your chest. Drop your knee toward the ground and catch hold of your left foot with your left hand. Take a big inhale and press your foot into your hand as you reach your opposite arm up for your dancer pose. Bend your knees and hug your shin back into your chest and place your foot back down.

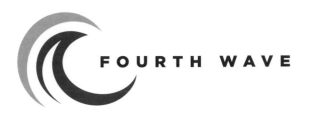

FOURTH WAVE

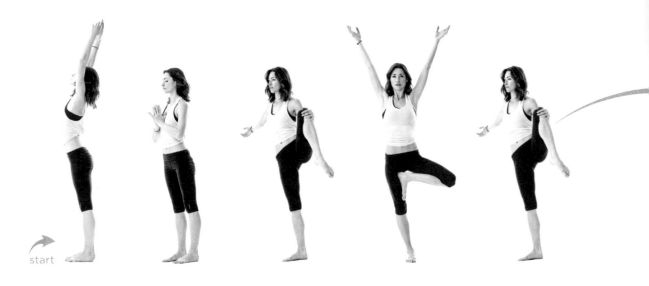

start

Take a big inhale and reach your arms up. Bring your palms together and bring your thumbs to your heartbeat. Close your eyes and see if you can feel your heart pumping.

Shift your weight onto your right leg; hug your left shin into your chest. Bring the bottom of your foot onto your thigh so your knee points out. Reach your arms up. Try closing your eyes and see how that changes your balance. Stay easy here like a tree swaying in the breeze. Hug your shin into your chest and bring your foot back down.

Repeat on the other side.

Shift your weight onto your right leg; hug your left shin into your chest. Wrap your left leg around your right and your left arm under your right for your eagle pose. Sink through your hips and lift up through your fingertips. Try with your eyes

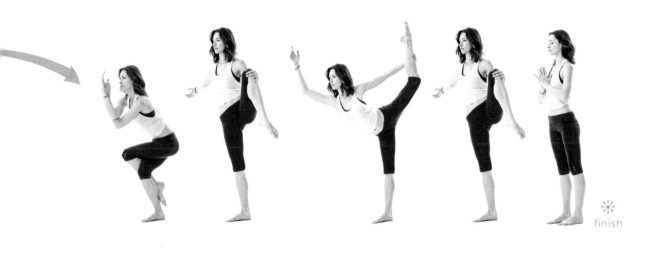

finish

closed to see how that changes your balance. Unwind out and hug your left shin back into your chest. Place your foot back down.

Repeat on the other side.

Shift your weight onto your right leg; hug your left shin into your chest. Drop your knee toward the ground and catch hold of your left foot with your left hand. Take a big inhale and press your foot into your hand as you reach your opposite arm up for your dancer pose. Try with your eyes closed to see how that changes your balance. Bend your knees and hug your shin back into your chest and place your foot back down.

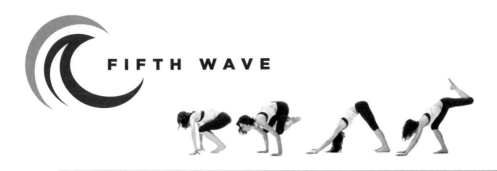

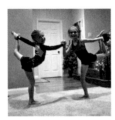
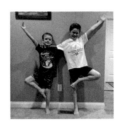
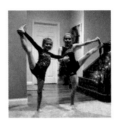

For crow show the movements and then take the time to go and help the kids who need an extra boost or tip to work on the movement. Same routine of demonstrating, then helping for handstand. Keep in mind these are really energetic, and the kids will probably get excited and be having fun. It's your job as the Guide to keep everyone safe while they try the movements. Use your instincts when you've given enough time to play around and when it's time to move on to the partner move. Bring up a volunteer to help demonstrate the partner move. Take the time to demonstrate it clearly with your partner, and then let everyone give it a try with a partner. Having them change partners a few times is a nice idea also. This is the big climax of the class, so take the time to go around and show support and encouragement as you help them get into the movements.

Come into a squat. Lean back, bringing your hands behind you. Take a big inhale and lean all the way forward, pressing your palms on the ground. Bring your knees around your arms. Look forward and lean forward. Exhale, come back, and relax. Try this a few times forward and back and side to side.

Come into your down dog. Walk your feet a little closer to your hands. Take a big inhale and lift your left leg up. Lean forward and rock forward a bit taking a little hop. Exhale, come back, and relax. Try this a few times on each side.

With your partner, grab hands, and hold on to your opposite ankle. Press your foot into your hand and use your partner for support for your dancer pose. Try both sides.

With your partner, grab hands, and bring your opposite foot into your thigh for your tree pose. Use your partner for support. Try both sides.

With your partner, grab hands, and grab hold of your opposite heel. Take a big inhale, and stretch your leg out to your side. Use your partner for support. Try both sides.

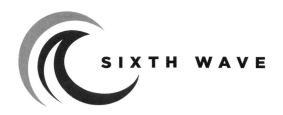

SIXTH WAVE

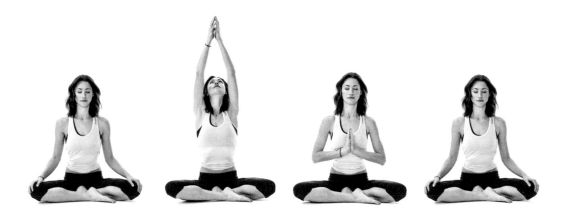

This is nice to demonstrate facing and mirroring the group to bring everyone back together with the breath and finish the class. Applause at the end is usually really fun and encouraging and a nice way to end after the breaths.

Sit comfortably. Take a big inhale and lift your arms out and up. Press your palms together and bring your thumbs to your heartbeat. Take a big inhale through your nose. Long exhale out through your mouth. Twice more like that. Big inhale. Long exhale. One more time. Big inhale. Long exhale. Relax your hands on your thighs and open your eyes. Great job everyone!

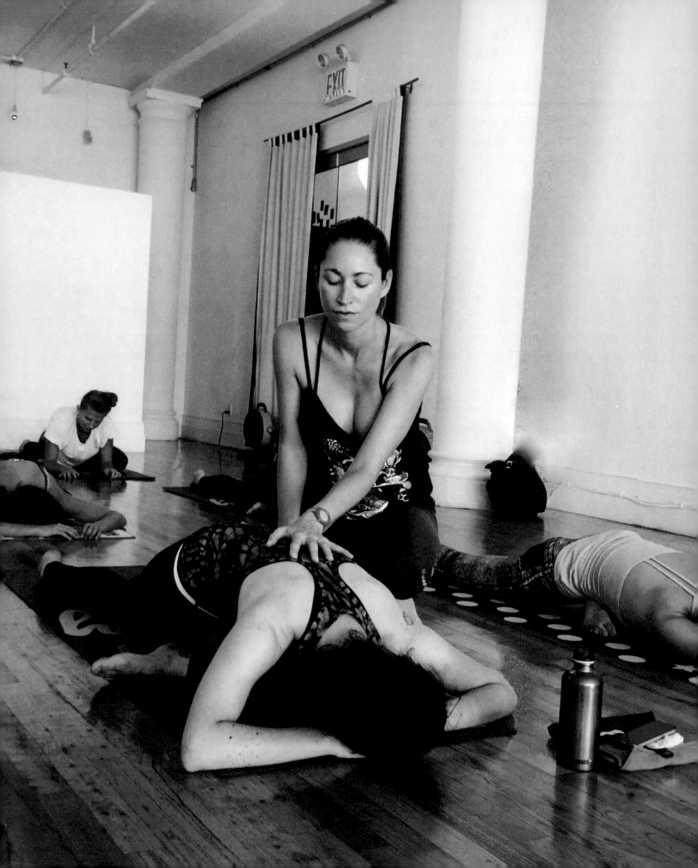

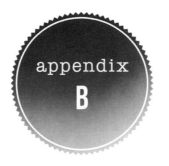

appendix

B

HEALING BACK PAIN

Yoga can be good for all kinds of health challenges, including injuries, chronic pain, and sleeplessness, along with a whole host of ailments associated with stress and obesity. Done right, yoga can help you lose or gain weight if you need it, activate and support your body's healing process for injuries and chronic pain, and allow stress to leave your body and mind, setting you on your best track for optimal health. The trick is our cure is often not simply a pose prescription. Unsurprisingly, it's something a bit more holistic and unique to each individual. Of course, giving people poses to do, for things like back pain, injuries, or weight loss, might work on some people, some of the time. But we're aiming for something that works for nearly everyone, nearly all the time.

What helps most—for pain, energy, sleep, and immunity—is often less about what poses you do and more about how you move your body. Here's the general guide, which works for both prevention and cure: move easy, everything you've got, in every direction you can.

You don't need to worry about poses, correct ways of doing things, or pushing into anything at all. From a health and healing perspective, it's best for you to stay relaxed, breathe deeply, and follow how you feel. It's not the poses that matter; it's you. So explore gently around and get to know all of you. When you find a place that feels good to linger, linger and breathe there! When you want to move, move easy.

There's also a great principle known as "surrounding the dragon." Dragons are very large, have big claws, and breathe fire. So attacking them head-on is rarely a wise idea. Instead you should carefully surround your dragons. Get to know them in this way, and you might even relax and make friends with them. You might also relax and make friends with yourself. This is where the healing principle comes in. When it comes to injuries, direct attacks on the injured area, like massage or rolling on balls, don't often help. Digging into an injury might sometimes feel good temporarily, but it rarely creates lasting gains.

Instead surround your dragon. Move softly around an injury. Lean just a little weight into it, and then release, allowing it to relax completely. Use hot-water bottles to complement this technique for promoting circulation and relaxation. You'll help stress leave the affected area and encourage your body to switch from defense into healing mode. This means trading stress for ease. Your body can stop defending itself against attack or additional pain and realign itself—both structurally and physiologically—for healing.

LOVING YOUR BACK

Chronic back pain is one of the most common challenges for people the world over. It's also an area where Western medicine often struggles. At times surgery seems like the only option, but the challenge with surgery is the two-year efficacy rate is almost the same as doing nothing.

Whether you get surgery or not, intervene with drugs or not, at some point you have to figure out how to help your body heal itself. You are the single most important participant in your own health and healing. From a surgeon's perspective, the back surgery is done, so it's a success! But for the person who had the surgery, recovery is long and painful, and lots of people wind up right back where they started two years later.

So take care of your back, whether it's about healing a current pain or preventing a future one, there are some simple things you can do. With a little knowledge and care, we can support our bodies to do what they like to do best: be healthy and feel good.

Following are steps you can take that will mobilize and stabilize your back, prevent injury, and stimulate healing as needed.

1. **RELAX! Avoid doing things that make you tense or rigid. Instead, do things that let stress release and leave your body and mind.**

2. **MOVE EASY, EVERYTHING YOU'VE GOT, IN EVERY DIRECTION YOU CAN MOVE IT. This creates the optimal conditions for triggering your body's healing response, and preventing onset of pain. Stay soft and movable in everything you do. If your body feels stiff and tense, find another way. There's always another way.**
   While you're moving, breathe extra deeply, so you can feel what you're moving through. When you find spots where it feels good to linger and breathe, linger and breathe. The moving and exploring is so you can find all the good spots. When you find them, stay a while. Scan through your body, find where you're holding tense as a response to

the pain, and let it go. It's not the easiest thing to relax when you're in pain, but it's important for shifting your body from defense into healing mode.

3. **DO THESE SIX EXERCISES** as often as you can during your day. This is where we get back specific.

    1) **Bridge lifts, three times, 10-second holds.** Lie on your back with your feet on the ground, knees up. Lift your hips up a few inches into a soft bridge, and squeeze your butt for 10 seconds! Release back down, rest, and repeat.

    2) **Scissor switch, 30 times.** Lie on your back, start with legs straight up, then scissor-switch (legs alternate straight up and down toward ground). Keep your knees soft and your lower back firmly connected to the ground (if it lifts up, just don't lower your feet as close to the ground).

    3) **Broken scissors, 30 times.** Start with legs straight up, open to sides and alternate crossing at upper thighs. Keep your knees soft.

    4) **Leg raises, 20 times.** Start with legs straight up. Lower toward the floor, then lift them until your hips lift and your lower back rounds slightly into the ground. Keep your knees soft.

    5) **Twist left and right, one to two minutes each side.** This can be an eagle twist or knee across body. Play around with how close you bring your crossing thigh to your body.

    6) **Crazy cat cow.** Now flip over onto your hands and knees and get comfortable, hands wider than your shoulders, knees wider than your hips. This is just a starting point. Now let your head hang easy, relax, and roll your hips and body around in every explorable direction. Rather than holding your arms stiff, let your elbows bend. Lean your hips over to one side, maybe far to one side as your calves swing around to the other side for balance. As you roll around left and right, ease your hips back toward your heels, then forward toward the ground. Your hands can move, your knees and feet can move, your ribs might round off

to one side or the other, a leg might extend daringly off to one side! Just keep moving from your belly, and let the rest of your body go along for the ride.

To help with all this movement, breathe! Breathe extra deeply, and hold a moment at the top of each breath, so you get to feel into everything you've got. You explore to find new spots in you where it feels good to linger and breathe. When you find them, linger and breathe! Let your breath take over. Use it even more than your muscles to get into your body here.

4. **WALK ON ALL FOURS.** This one people don't usually listen to, until they're really in pain! Interestingly enough, this works really well for everyone I know who has used it. Walk around on all fours—hands and knees—every morning when you're first getting out of bed, and every night before you go back to bed. Do this for at least a few minutes each time. Amazingly, it has a way of "moving easily, everything you've got, in every direction" that helps regenerate your body's natural support structure and alignment along your spine.

5. **USE HEAT.** Get two hot-water bottles, fill them with hot water straight from your tap—not scalding, just warm in a way that feels good—and surround whatever hurts. This doesn't always mean putting the bottle right on an injury. When part of your back hurts, a fairly extended area can become stiff and tense as part of your body's defensive reaction. Explore what feels good throughout your whole back, down into your hips, and up into your shoulders.

There you have it! A few things you can do to help your back feel better. Just remember these two things:

1. Do this every day! Your body responds really well to what you do, and what you don't do, every day.

2. Do all of this with ease. It should feel less like exercise and more like getting into your body.

LOVING THE REST OF YOU

The same principles that we discussed at the beginning of this section aren't back specific. They can be applied to shoulders, wrists, hips, and knees.

While not as common as back pain, chronic pain and tenderness often spring up for people in their hips and shoulders. Poses like hip and shoul-

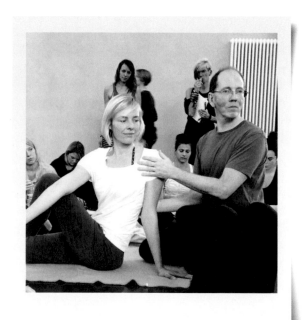

der openers can feel quite good while you're doing them, but over time, pushing farther into these poses creates hypermobility in most people, which leads to more pain. So it's not another pose that's likely to help here. To restore balance in your body, put your focus on moving rather than posing. In fact, forget the pose altogether if it causes any pain.

Wrists are another joint that frequently becomes painful for people who practice a lot of yoga. The most common cause here is jumping forward from down dog, and jumping back to plank from forward folds. This sudden movement pits the strength of your thighs against your wrists. Eventually your wrists lose. The fix here is often equally straightforward. Unlike your more complicated knee and shoulder joints, wrists frequently heal quite rapidly when you simply stop jumping and move easily instead. If some help is needed, two hot-water bottles twice each day on your wrists and forearms can relax the surrounding area, promote helpful circulation, and set your body on the right track for healing.

Overall, just keep moving your body easily all around every pose—over, under, left, right, forward, back, up, and down. Let your body relax. Don't use force to get into anything. Just explore gently in every direction. Rather than bringing stress into your body and mind, this will help send it in the direction you want: right on out of you. Once your mind and body feel safe, your critical systems can switch from defense mode into healing and happy mode.

Your body is an incredible healing machine, and it will often just take care of itself with a little time. Our bodies are pretty great that way. If you want to support that healing process, even better.

Far from lazy, this kind of moving and exploration has a way of making people supercapable in their own bodies. The best part is, you get great at being in you. You've made friends with you! From here, your body can get to work, drawing on its own incredible capacity to heal and live radiant and happy. From here, you are your own best cure.

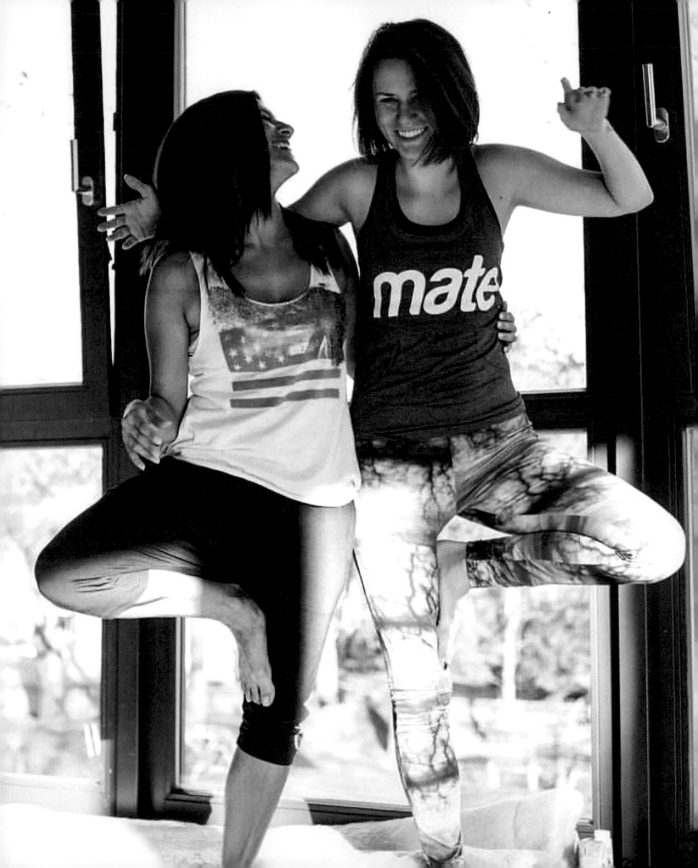

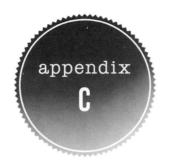

PROTECTING & HEALING YOUR KNEES

Your knees are amazing! The knee is an incredible piece of engineering, structured as a "pivotal hinge joint." This means it not only swings back and forth, but also has a slight rotational capacity, allowing you to navigate easily over uneven ground. It also has a highly advanced system of lubricating fluid and cushioning sacks to keep things protected and moving easily. What's extraspecial about this protective fluid is that it's not dumb. Land hard from a jump, and it instantly becomes more viscous to absorb shock. Lighten your load and viscosity immediately reduces to support easy movement.

Of course, complicated engineering can be vulnerable. If you play sports, carry heavy loads, or just live your life for a bit, you've probably noticed that knees don't always feel great. They can also take quite a long time to heal, so when your knees send you signals, it's important to listen!

The number one way to prevent injury: if something hurts your knee, don't do it. Find another way. There's always a way to do what you need to do that feels good.

If you have some knee pain or an injury, it's a great idea to talk with your doctor about these things. It helps to have direct advice from someone qualified, who knows your particular case history. From here, I can share from our experience at Strala, and my background in mind-body medicine.

Moving is good. Not so long ago, the medical approach to injury was to immobilize us for a long time. This kept people from hurting themselves even worse, but it made rehab long and challenging, and often inhibited complete recovery.

Now, whenever possible, maintaining mobility is a more common treatment path. You want to support your body's natural healing process. Your body is great! But it can use your help. In general, you can support yourself by moving easy, everything you've got, in every direction you can. (Sound familiar?)

In this case "moving easy" means not putting much extra weight or stress on the knee. You don't want the injury or surrounding areas to feel challenged or strained. Yoga poses aren't particularly crucial here, and you especially don't want to "stretch" your knee in any way. If you're a yoga person interested in knee safety, dropping hero poses and not pushing into hip openers is always a good idea.

Instead to restore and maintain healthy balance and mobility, you want to move easy. This is a great practice to drop tension out of your body, support healing, and build a healthy state of well-being. To stay easygoing, lie on your back and hold one thigh with both hands, so your knee is about vertical over your hip. Relax, and let your calf just hang easy. Then gently wiggle your thigh with your hands, so your calf softly rolls around and swings side to side. Explore different hand, arm, thigh, and whole-body positions, to find what feels most relaxed, and what makes it easiest to move without strain. Open the hip off to the side for a bit; then bring it across your body for a twist. Support your thigh as you extend your leg straight up, keeping the knee and leg relaxed—not stiff or stick-straight—and just give the whole leg a little wiggle and roll-around. These are all starting points. You get to find what feels best for you each day. There's lots of freedom to explore here, so use it and explore!

What you want to avoid is putting stress on your knee. If something hurts, don't do it! Find a way that doesn't hurt. When you're in pain, it puts stress into your body and mind. From here, the body kicks into defense mode. This is great for preventing an even worse injury, but it's not great for healing. To heal, you need to relax! Let stress leave your body. You can do this by finding places that you're comfortable, and moving gently from them.

Remember that going easy is far from going lazy. So it doesn't mean ignore the injury and just lie around! It means move all around it, finding places that feel good to linger and breathe, and lingering and breathing right there. Moving evenly around an injury in this relaxed way has mechanical benefits of relaxing the surrounding areas and improving local circulation. It also triggers your body's relaxation response.

One last tip: hot-water bottles! Use two of them, filled with hot water from your tap. Explore what feels good up your thigh and into your lower back, as well as down into your calf.

Give your body a little support, and it will continue to perform miracles for you. Let me know how it goes!

INDEX

ACKNOWLEDGMENTS

Laura Gray, thank you for your understanding of Strala and tireless help with wrapping this all together in a sensible and useful way. Forever thank you to Patty Gift, Reid Tracy, Sally Mason-Swaab, Richelle Fredson, and the entire Hay House family for making space for this work and for your mentorship and countless lessons and patience.

Charles McStravick, you're a visual dream and I'm so lucky to have you bring the vibrancy and energy of the Strala community to life on these pages. Thank you!

Sam Berlind, thank you for being such an integral part of the Strala Leadership Programs and bringing your experience and passion to all we do together.

Mike, it's almost silly to continue to thank you since we are a package deal at this point. Working with your partner is something that freaks out many, but magically we evolved to having THE BEST TIME ever and always.

Kayleigh Pleas, your six second hugs, and lessons in compassion and self-care are extraordinary, and thank you always for your contributions to the Strala community.

Dr. Rudy Tanzi, and Deepak Chopra, thank you for your endless support, friendship, and guidance on how I can better serve. I'm eternally grateful for your collaboration.

Rory Foster and Kendall DuVay, thank you for your guidance and friendship over the years. I wouldn't have the pleasure to do what I do without your teaching and care.

To all the Strala Guides, studio owners, managers, supporters, and helpers around the world, this book, this work, this process evolves out of the joy of each of you. Thank you for your endless excitement, ease, attention, and thoughtful leadership you bring to yourself and those you reach. You are helping the world in so many ways, it's incredible and impossible to quantify.

To all who practice with us from around the world, you're everywhere and radiating all the good vibes! We love you loads and are incredibly grateful and humble you find this work and process of ease useful. Please always let us know how we can be better for you.

Jason and Colleen Wachob, thank you for your friendship, support, and always being there.

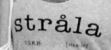

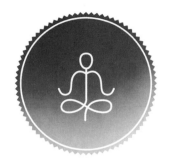

ABOUT THE AUTHOR

TARA STILES is the founder and owner of Strala, a revolutionary approach to healing through movement. Thousands of Guides lead Strala classes around the globe in partner studios, gyms, and clubs. Strala has been illustrated in a case study by Harvard Business School, and its philosophy of ease and conservation of energy are incorporated by business leaders, entrepreneurs, and well-being professionals around the world.

Tara teams up with W Hotels, bringing Strala Yoga and healthy recipes to W properties around the globe. She is a collaborator with Reebok, working closely with the design team on their Reebok Yoga lifestyle range, and has authored several best-selling books, including *Yoga Cures*, *Make Your Own Rules Cookbook*, and *Strala Yoga*, all translated and published in several different languages. She has been profiled by *The New York Times*, *Times of India*, *The Times (UK)*, and featured in most major national and international magazines.

Tara supports the Alliance for a Healthier Generation, President Clinton's initiative to combat childhood obesity, bringing Strala classes to 30,000-plus participating schools. Tara is married to Mike Taylor. They live in SOHO with their daughter.

Visit stralayoga.com.

MIKE TAYLOR is the co-founder of Strala and known

for leading the science and movement of the programs. Mike studied mind-body medicine at Harvard and complementary medicine at Oxford. He has

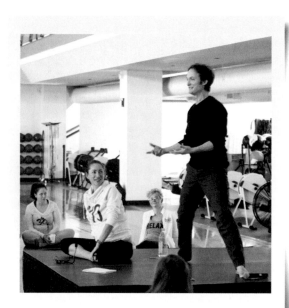

practiced Eastern movement and healing, including tai chi and qigong, for 30 years.

In his younger years, Mike challenged centuries of reasonable and well-tested martial traditions in hundreds of competitions, by applying unruly imagination to a world where rules were unbreakable. His record established the strength of finding your own way in your own body, rather than copying the techniques of other people's traditions. As he got older, he continued on to medical applications of the mind-body connection in university. After running into walls with standard medical practice in the United States and England, Mike left his health-care roots. He worked at a steel mill for a while, joined a web company, and then founded a few more.

Now Mike has found his way back to health care done right, helping people let go of stress in their bodies and minds, and become their own best caregivers. Mike climbs mountains in his spare time. He is married to Tara Stiles. They live in SOHO with their daughter.

SAM BERLIND is an Ohashiatsu teacher & practitioner living in New York City. While studying comparative religion and philosophy at the University of Edinburgh in 1981, he began to practice Iyengar yoga, and he has continued to practice and teach yoga after moving to New York.

Eager to learn more about the relationship between the healing properties of yoga and traditional Asian medicine, he began studying with Wataru Ohashi. Sam fell in love with shiatsu, began teaching Ohashiatsu in 1987, and led the Ohashiatsu school in New York for 20 years. He has since taught in New York, Omega Institute, and throughout the United States and Europe.

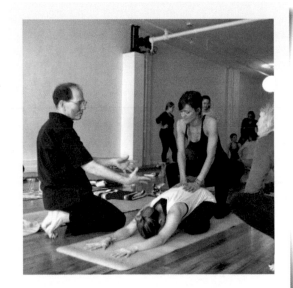

Sam also teaches enhancement workshops and seminars based on his study of Feldenkrais Method, Gestalt therapy, Zen Shiatsu, TCM, and other modalities. His understanding of the healing arts is deeply influenced by his study and teaching of martial arts since 1988. Sam has been collaborating with Strala since 2010.

HAY HOUSE TITLES

OF

RELATED INTEREST

YOU CAN HEAL YOUR LIFE, the movie,
starring **LOUISE HAY & FRIENDS**

(available as a 1-DVD program and an expanded 2-DVD set)
Watch the trailer at: www.LouiseHayMovie.com

THE SHIFT, the movie,
starring **DR. WAYNE W. DYER**

(available as a 1-DVD program and an expanded 2-DVD set)
Watch the trailer at: www.DyerMovie.com

• • •

Light Is the New Black:
A Guide to Answering Your Soul's Callings and Working Your Light,
BY REBECCA CAMPBELL

Perfectly Imperfect: The Art and Soul of Yoga Practice,
BY BARON BAPTISTE

You Have 4 Minutes to Change Your Life: Simple 4-Minute Meditations for
Inspiration, Transformation, and True Bliss,
BY REBEKAH BORUCKI

Your 3 Best Super Powers: Meditation, Imagination & Intuition,
BY SONIA CHOQUETTE

All of the above are available at your local bookstore,
or may be ordered by contacting Hay House (see next page).